AF327279

# Art and Science of
# CLEFT LIP AND CLEFT PALATE REPAIR

# Art and Science of
# CLEFT LIP AND CLEFT PALATE REPAIR


**Girish N Amlani**
MS (General surgery) MCh (Plastic surgery)
Honorary Plastic Surgeon
Shri NM Virani Wockhardt Hospital, Rajkot
Sterling Hospital, Sri HJ Doshi
General Hospital, Shri GT Seth Orthopaedic
Hospital, Gokul Hospital, Rajkot and
Gokul Newtech Hospital, Jamnagar
Mahatma Gandhi Institute of Medical Sciences
Vardha, Ramkrishna Sahyadri Hospital
Gandhidham and Wockhardt Hospital
Bhavnagar, Gujarat, India


*Foreword*
**Santosh Raibagkar**

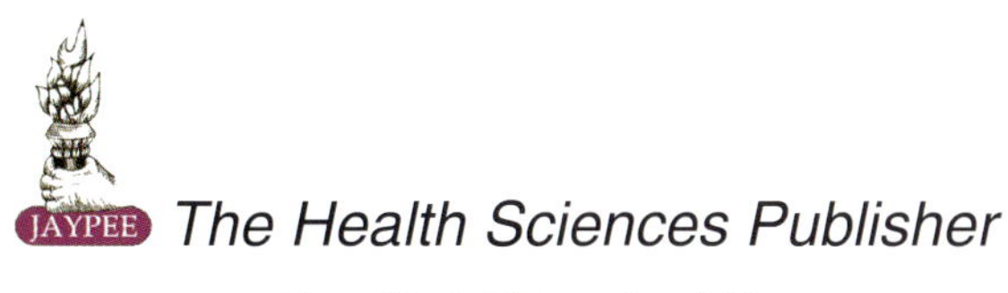

*The Health Sciences Publisher*
New Delhi | London | Panama

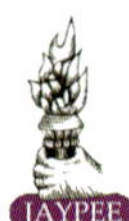

**Jaypee Brothers Medical Publishers (P) Ltd**

**Headquarters**

Jaypee Brothers Medical Publishers (P) Ltd
4838/24, Ansari Road, Daryaganj
New Delhi 110 002, India
Phone: +91-11-43574357
Fax: +91-11-43574314
Email: jaypee@jaypeebrothers.com

**Overseas Offices**

J.P. Medical Ltd
83 Victoria Street, London
SW1H 0HW (UK)
Phone: +44 20 3170 8910
Fax: +44 (0)20 3008 6180
Email: info@jpmedpub.com

Jaypee Brothers Medical Publishers (P) Ltd
17/1-B Babar Road, Block-B, Shaymali
Mohammadpur, Dhaka-1207
Bangladesh
Mobile: +08801912003485
Email: jaypeedhaka@gmail.com

Jaypee-Highlights Medical Publishers Inc
City of Knowledge, Bld. 235, 2nd Floor Clayton
Panama City, Panama
Phone: +1 507-301-0496
Fax: +1 507-301-0499
Email: cservice@jphmedical.com

Jaypee Brothers Medical Publishers (P) Ltd
Bhotahity, Kathmandu, Nepal
Phone: +977-9741283608
Email: kathmandu@jaypeebrothers.com

Website: www.jaypeebrothers.com
Website: www.jaypeedigital.com



*Art and Science of Cleft Lip and Cleft Palate Repair*

*First Edition*: **2017**
ISBN 978-93-86150-59-2
*Printed at* Replika Press Pvt. Ltd.

### Dedicated to
*My parents, teachers and family members*

# Foreword

I feel great pleasure to write the foreword for the book *Art and Science of Cleft Lip and Palate Repair*. I know Girish Amlani since 1993 when he joined SCL Hospital as a MCh (Plastic surgery) Registrar. He is very sincere and hard working and has skilled surgical hands.

The book has excellent description of all the aspects of cleft lip and cleft palate. It has excellent illustrations of very important surgical steps. This book will be very useful to students of plastic surgery.

**Santosh Raibagkar**
MS MCh (Plastic surgery)
Professor and Head
AMC MET Medical College
LG General Hospital
Ahmedabad, Gujarat
India

# Preface

The legendary late Dr Udayan H Vyas, Ex-Professor and Head of the Department of Plastic Surgery Unit, SCL Hospital, Ahmedabad, Gujarat, India had great interest in cleft lip and palate surgery. Dr Santosh C Raibagkar, Professor and Head of the Department of Plastic Surgery Unit AMC MET Medical College and LG General Hospital, Ahmedabad, an Associate Professor at that time had great interest in facial plastic surgery. They gave me dissertation of "A study of 40 cases—Hegarty's unilateral cleft lip repair" in 1993–1995. The thought of the paper is being elaborated in the book format. In this book, embryology and anatomy of cleft lip and cleft palate is very interesting. Various classification systems have been mentioned with clinical photographs. Unilateral cleft lip repair, bilateral cleft lip repair, cleft palate repair, cleft nose repair, operation for velopharyngeal insufficiency are described with drawings and photographs. Guidelines for anesthesia in cleft surgeries help reduce mortality and mortalities associated with cleft surgeries.

**Girish N Amlani**

# Acknowledgments

I express deep sense of gratitude to my respected teacher late Dr Udayan H Vyas, Ex-Professor and Head of the Department of Plastic Surgery Unit, SCL Hospital, Ahmedabad, Gujarat, India.

I am greatly indebted to Dr Santosh C Raibagkar, Professor and Head of Department of Plastic Surgery Unit, AMC MET Medical College, LG General Hospital, Ahmedabad, Gujarat, India.

I thank Khorakiwala Family, especially Ms Zahabiya Khorakiwala, Managing Director of Wockhardt Group of Hospitals for running Smile Train Program for more than 10 years. The trustees of Shri Ashok Gondhia Memorial Trust and Management of NM Virani Wockhardt Hospitals were very helpful. I thank the anesthetist team, especially Dr Rajesh Radadia, Dr Dhaval Karoriya, Dr Tejas Chauhan, Dr Rajesh Sakaria, Dr Khyati Purohit and to the pediatrician team, especially Dr Mehul Mitra and Dr Trupti Vaishnani for taking excellent care.

I especially thank Mr Satish Kalra (Chief Programme Officer), Mrs Mamta Carrol (Regional Director India), Mrs Renu Mehta (Country Director, India) of Smile Train Programme.

I thank Shri Jitendra P Vij (Group Chairman), Mr Ankit Vij (Group President), Mr KK Raman, Mr DC Gupta, Mrs Priyanka Kansara and Mr Sharad Patel of M/s Jaypee Brothers Medical Publishers (Pvt) Ltd, New Delhi, India for their constant support and help in publishing this book.

The most outstanding contribution was the cooperation of the parents of my patients born with congenital deformities.

# Contents

# CHAPTER 1

# Historical Perspective

## HISTORY OF CLEFT LIP

Cleft lips have been present from time immemorial, but the attitude and reaction of society have been varied greatly. It has been said that in certain societies, a cleft was once considered a mark of beauty. However, in other eras, cleft children were not so fortunate, and in accord with certain tribal customs, all deformed children were discarded or sacrificed.

An unnamed Chinese surgeon repaired a cleft lip in 4th century AD. The result must have been reasonably successful since his patient, Wei Yang-Chi, became a Governor-general of six Chinese provinces.[1]

The early surgery consisted of simple denudation of the cleft lip edge, and a V-excision as described in the Saxon Leech Book of Bald, written in the later part of the 10th century.

In 13th century Europe, Jehan Yperman, a Flemish surgeon described repair of cleft lips. Ambroise Paré (1510–1590) discussed closure of cleft lip with needles and wax threads which were wrapped around the ends of the needle in figure of eight fashion (Fig. 1.1).

Velpeau (1839) stated that Celsus and other ancient surgeons in addition to paring harelips made relaxing incisions on the inner surface of the cheek prior to suturing.

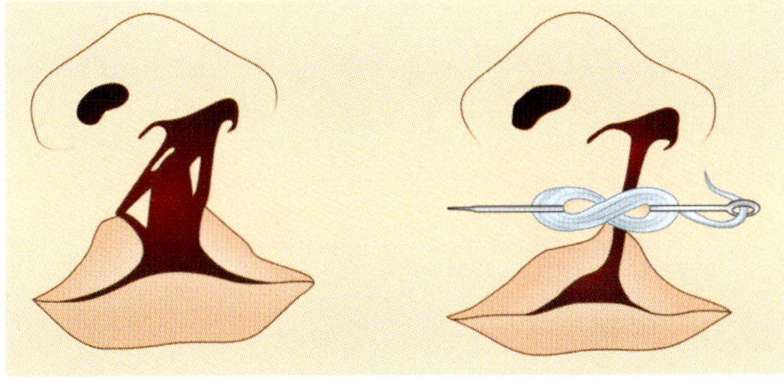

**Fig. 1.1:** Ambroise Paré (1510–1590) described closure of cleft lip with needles and wax threads

Franco (1561) is also credited with recommending freeing of the soft part of the cheek from the maxilla prior to closure.[2]

A step forward from the simple paring of cleft edges (actually a V-excision) several men recommended curving or angulating the denuding incision, thus providing for increasing length of the sutured lip. Graefe in 1825 attempted to overcome subsequence notching by curving this incision.

Mirault of Anger,[3] France 1844, described repair of total cleft lip and partial cleft lip by turning down tiny vermilion flaps from either side of the cleft and then cutting one of them off where he approximated the edges. Mirault when wrote his original paper, had woodcuts which poorly illustrated this technique (Fig. 1.2A).

In 1891, Rose of London employed curved incision from the nostril floor to the vermilion border of the lip so as to give a line of union sufficiently long yet not discarding good tissue at the mucocutaneous line (Fig. 1.2B). Thompson in 1912 described a similar curving of the incised wound edges, first making careful and accurate measurements with calipers (Fig. 1.2C).

In order to prevent contraction of the postoperative scar, several methods were devised which resulted in an irregularly outlined scar. The procedure described by Owen (1904) resulted in an angulated scar running laterally. Unfortunately much of the lateral vermilion border was discarded.

The Koenig operation (1898) also introduced tissue from the medial side of the cleft laterally.

It had become apparent to other surgeons[4-6] that instead of moving inadequate medial tissue laterally, a transplanting of some of the full lateral tissues into the deficient medial portion of the cleft was desirable. Hagedorn

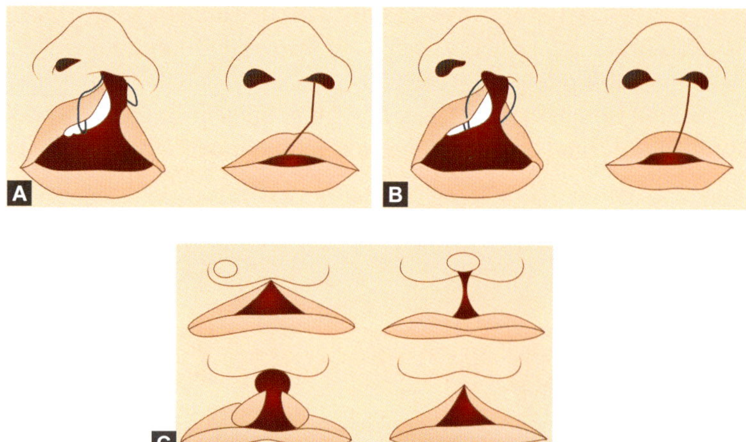

**Figs 1.2A to C:** (A) Mirault (1844) described repair of total cleft lip and partial cleft lip by turning down tiny vermilion flaps; (B) Rose (1891) employed curved incision from nostril floor to vermilion border of the lip; (C) Thompson (1912) described a similar curving of incised wound edges, first making measurement with calipers

in 1892 described a procedure which had been considered the forerunner of the present day rectangular flap. This procedure produced a desirable fullness at the vermilion border. Veau in his Bec De Lievre (1938) gave credit to Jalanguier who in 1910 described and illustrated a procedure bringing some lateral tissue to the area of the deficiency medially. As noted in his illustrations, however, he discarded more mucous membrane from the lateral portion of the lip than one would do today.[7-9]

Blair and Brown in their original article in 1930 described a lateral flap, one-half length of the lip. To these authors went the credit for insistence upon production of pouting lip in these infants. They also paid attention to the correction of the deformed nostril.

About this time Lemesurier[10-12] of Toronto became aware of the possibilities of modification of the Hagedorn principle for some 13 years before presenting this work in 1948 (Fig. 1.3).

The Tennison method,[13,14] using a triangular flap originally outlined with a bent wire stencil, was introduced in 1952 that impressed many surgeons with its good cosmetic results and its relative simplicity. One of its selling point was preservation of normal looking cupid's bow on the medial lip segment, a landmark, largely ignored before (Fig. 1.4).

Marks in 1953 further clarified the techniques of the triangular flap but essentially along Tennison's line.[14] Randall (1959)[15] and Hegarty 1958 have added modification of the triangular flap insert (Figs 1.5 and 1.6). Skoog[16] 1958 described the breaking up straight line by introduction to smaller triangles giving credit in principle to Trauner and Gillies.

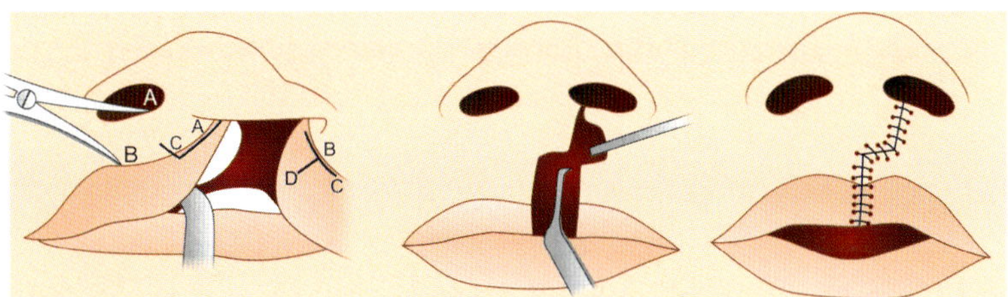

**Fig. 1.3:** Lemesurier (1940) described rectangular flap from full lateral tissue into the deficient medial portion of the cleft

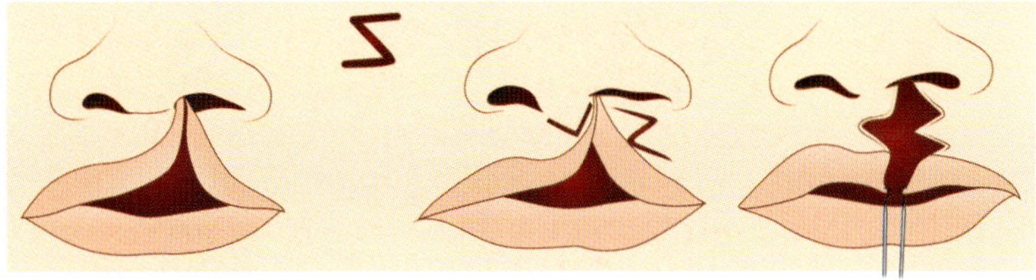

**Fig. 1.4:** Tennison (1952) used a bent wire stencil to outline incisions

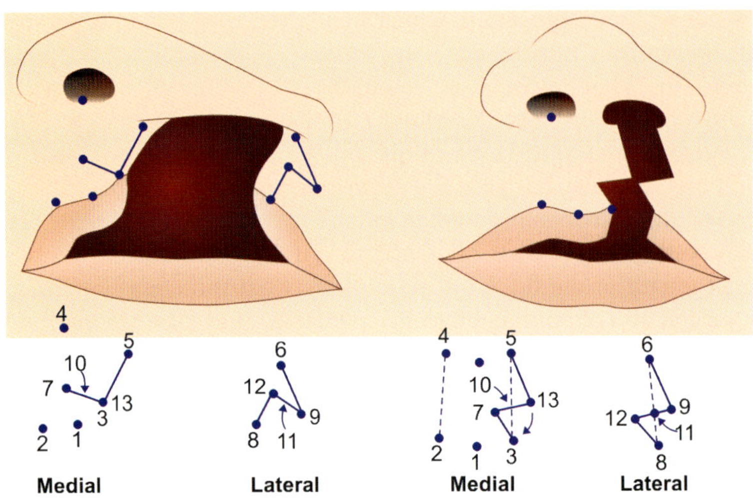

**Fig. 1.5:** Randall (1958) added modification of the triangular flap insert

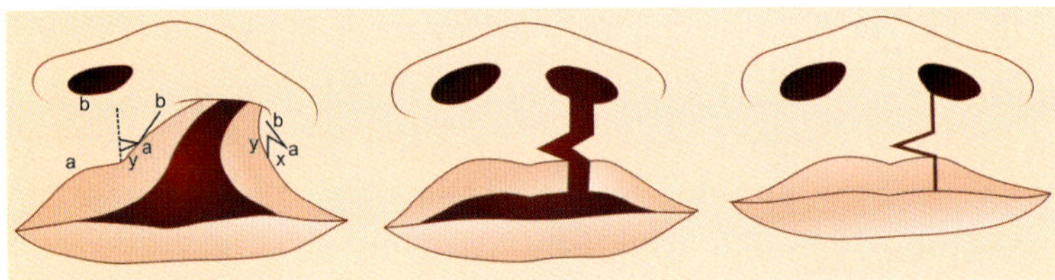

**Fig. 1.6:** Hegarty's unilateral cleft lip repair (1958): Hegarty modified triangular flap technique. All points and incisions are based on mathematics

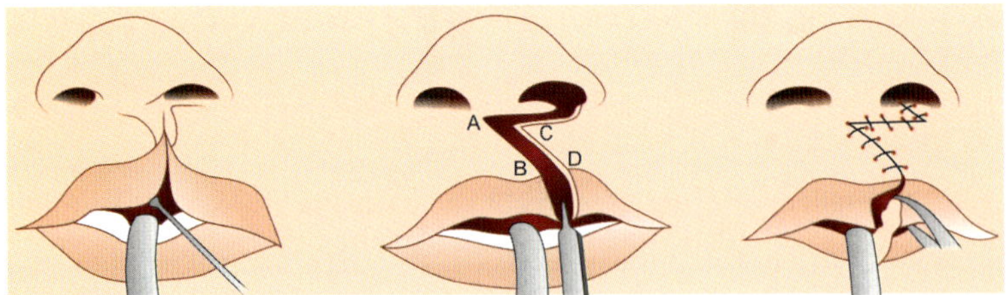

**Fig. 1.7:** Rotation and advancement technique introduced by Millard (1955): recolonized surgical lip repair

The rotation and advancement technique introduce by Millard[17] in 1955. The Millard rotation advancement technique revolutionized surgical lip repair (Fig. 1.7). The Z plasty type of scar thus produced is also evident in other lip repair (Fig. 1.8). Clifford and Pool (1959) review the Z plasty principles in cleft lip surgery.

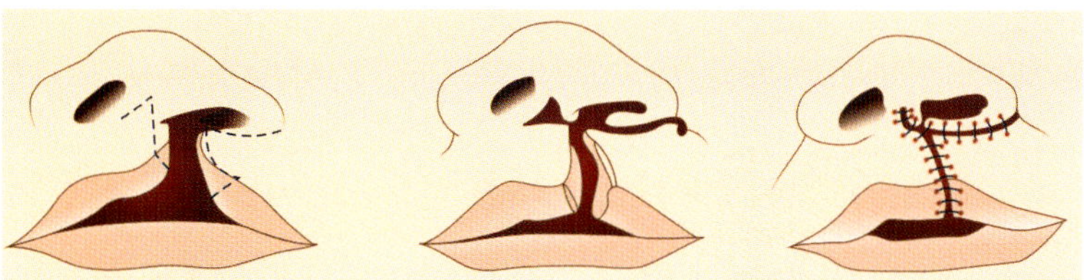

**Fig. 1.8:** Mohler (1986) modified rotation and advancement to produce scar line mimic normal philtrum column by extending rotation incision into the columella

## HISTORY OF CLEFT PALATE

Cleft palate was initially confused with defect caused by tertiary syphilis. In early 19th Century first cleft palate repair was done and with introducing of anesthesia cleft palate repair become common. Von Graefe was the first surgeon to perform cleft palate before 1819. Philibert Roux[18] described cleft palate repair around same time in Paris. John Collins Warren was first in America is report cleft palate repair in 1920 in Boston.

Dieffenback[19] (1792–1847), Berlin passed multiple silver or lead wires through punch holes to bring both palatal bones together. Von Lagenback[20] used bilateral mucoperiosteal flaps for cleft palate closure. Double opposite Z-plasty, Dorrence's pushback and veaus palatal muscles dissection are quite significant in recent times.[21]

## REFERENCES


1. Boo-chai K. An Ancient Chinese text on a cleft lip. Plast Reconstr Surg. 1966;38:89-91.
2. Barsky AJ. Pierre Franco, father of cleft lip surgery. His life and times. Br J Plast Surg. 1964;17:335-50.
3. Blair VP, Brown JB. Mirault operation for single hare lip. Surg Gyn Obstet. 1930;51:81.
4. Brown JB, McDowell F. Simplified design for repair of single cleft lip. Surg Gyn Obst. 1945;80:12-26.
5. Rogers BO. History of cleft lip and palate treatment. In: Grabb WC, (Ed). Cleft lip and palate. Boston: Little, Brown; 1971.
6. Washio H. History of cleft lip surgery. In: Stark RB (Ed). Cleft palate: A multidisciplinary approach, New York: Hoeber Medical Division. Harper and Row, 1968.
7. Schultz LW. Bilateral cleft lips. Plast Reconstr Surg. 1946;1:338-43.
8. Veau V. Operative treatment of complete double harelip. Ann Surg. 1922;76:143-56.
9. Veau V. Division Palatine. Paris: Masson, 1931.
10. Bauer TB, Trusler HM and Glanz S. Repair of unilateral cleft lip. Advantage of LeMesurier technique use of mucous membrane flap in maxillary clefts. Plast Reconstr Surg. 1953;11:56-8.
11. Le Mesurier AB. Hare-Lips and their Treatment. Baltimore: Williams and Wilkins. 1962:120-43.

12. LeMesurier AB. A method of cutting and suturing the lip in the treatment of complete unilateral clefts. Plastic Reconstr Surg. 1949;4(1):1-12.
13. Brauer RO. Comparison of Tennison's and LeMesurier technique of lip repair. Plast Reconstr Surg. 1959;23:249.
14. Tennison CW. The repair of unilateral cleft lip by stencil method. Plast Reconstr Surg. 1952;9:115-20.
15. Randall P. A triangular flap operation for primary repair of unilateral clefts of lip. Plast Reconstr Surg. 1959;23:331.
16. Skoog T. A design for repair of unilateral cleft lip. American Journal of Surgery. 1958;95:223-5.
17. Millard DR Jr. Rotation-advancement principle in cleft lip closure. Cleft Palate J. 1964;1:246-52.
18. Efin MA. Dr Roux's first operation of soft palate in 1819: A historical vignette. Cleft Palate Craniofac J. 1999;36:27-9.
19. Goldwyn RM, Johann Friedrich Dieffenback (1794–1847). Plast Reconstr Surg. 1968;42:19-28.
20. Goldwyn RM, Bernhard Van Lagenbeck. This life and legacy. Plast Reconstr Surg. 1969;44:248-54.
21. Stephenson J. Repair of cleft palate by Philibert Roux in 1819. Plast Reconstr Surg. 1971;47:277-83.

# CHAPTER 2

# Anesthesia

All patients are operated under general anesthesia[1-7] with endotracheal intubation. 24 G or 22 G intracath are used for itravenous access. Injection glycopyrrolate (0.004 mg/kg) intravenous (IV), injection Emeset (0.1 mg/kg) IV, injection paracetamol (10 mg/kg) IV with antibiotics are given as premedication.

Patients are induced with injection thiopentone (7 mg/kg) IV, injection scoline (2 mg/kg) IV. We avoid propofol below six months of age. Endotracheal tube (RAE) (Fig. 2.1) in pediatric age group and south oral tube in adults[8] are prefered.

Muscle relaxants are avoided in cleft lip cases while cleft palate patients are given atracurium 0.5 mg/kg IV. Patients are maintained in anesthesia with injection atracurium, sevoflurane, oxygen and nitrous oxide.[9,10]

Injection glycopyrrolate (0.006 mg/kg) and injection neostigmine (0.05 mg/kg) IV are used for reversal.

Postopratively patients are kept in either in lateral position or in semiprone position. We have to watch for bleeding postoperatively.[11]

Patients are kept nil orally for 4 hours preoperatively. Cow's milk and solid diet should be stopped before 6 hours of surgery. Patients can be given clear fluids like glucose water and apple juice before 4 hours of surgery.

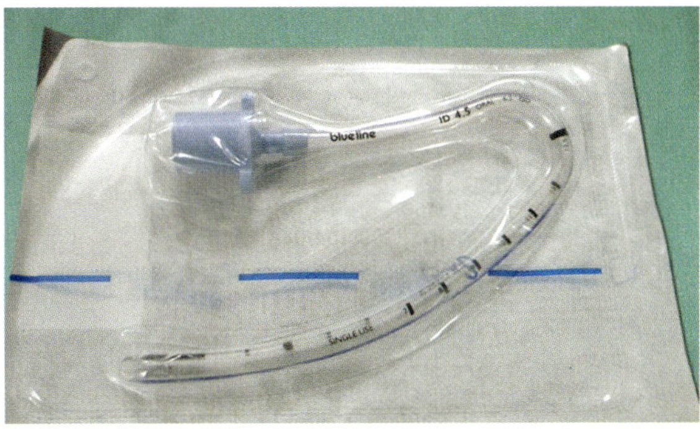

**Fig. 2.1:** Right angle endotracheal (RAE) tube

Patients kept nil orally for more than 4 hours before surgery can develop acute dehydration which can lead to serious consequences particularly in summer.

Hypotonic solution like Isolyte-P should be avoided during perioperative fluid therapy. Isolyte-P consists of 80% free water and becomes hypotonic once glucose is metabolized. Infusion of hypotonic solution can lead to iatrogenic hyponatremia leading to intractable seizures due to cerebral edema and encephalopathy. Patients weighing under 15 kg of weight should given fluid with micro drip set with 100 cc chamber or with infusion pump to avoid fluid overload. Measuring serum electrolyte and serum glucose level during perioperative period can be useful.

We use infraorbital nerve blocks[12,13] for unilateral and bilateral cleft lip surgeries (Figs 2.2 to 2.6) and suprazygomatic maxillary nerve block[14,15] (Figs 2.7 to 2.9) in pediatric patients and infrazygomatic maxillary nerve block (Figs 2.10 and 2.11) in adult patients for cleft palate surgeries preoperatively. Using regional anesthesia reduces complication during and after surgery and

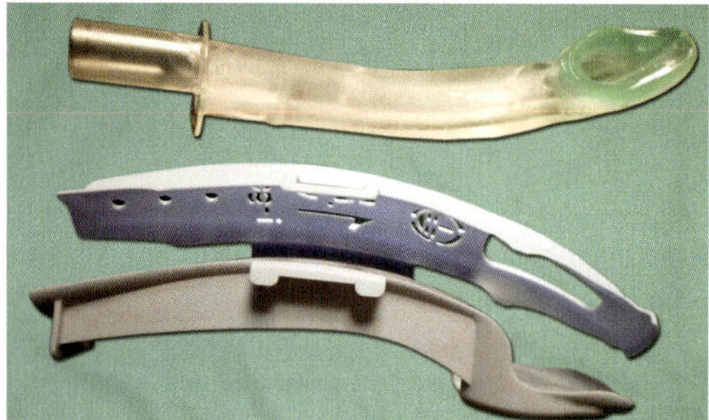

**Fig. 2.2:** I-gel: size 1: 2–5 kg, size 1.5: 5–12 kg, size 2.0: 10–25 kg, size 2.5: 25–35 kg

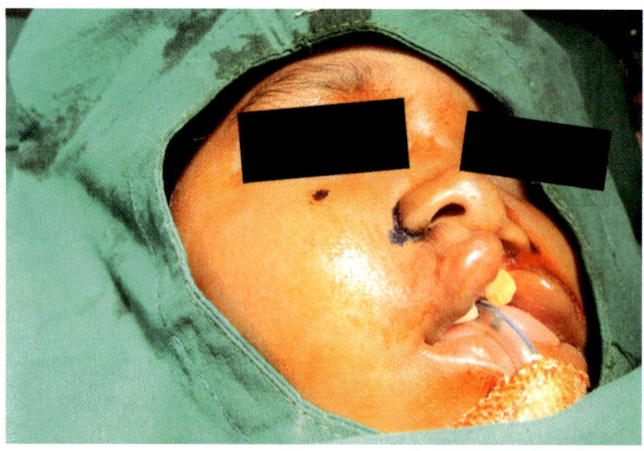

**Fig. 2.3:** Bilateral infraorbital nerve block:[12,13] Three points are marked over lateral canthus, lateral alar region and midpoint of both. Local anesthesia is given over midpoint just below infraorbital rim over infraorbital nerve

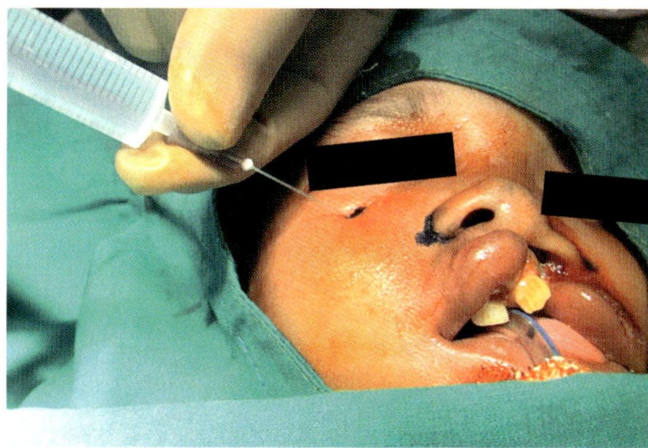

**Fig. 2.4:** Right infraorbital nerve block

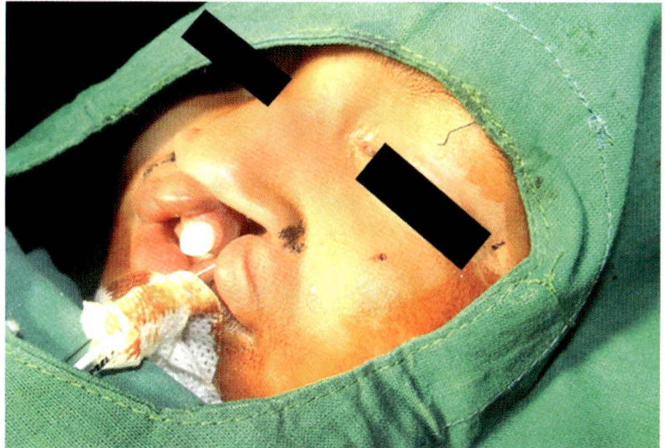

**Fig. 2.5:** Three points are marked A: Lateral alar region C: Lateral canthol region B: B midpoint of A and C

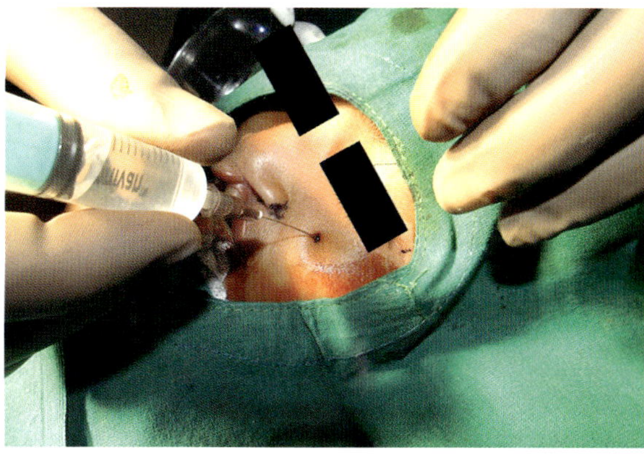

**Fig. 2.6:** Left infraorbital nerve block

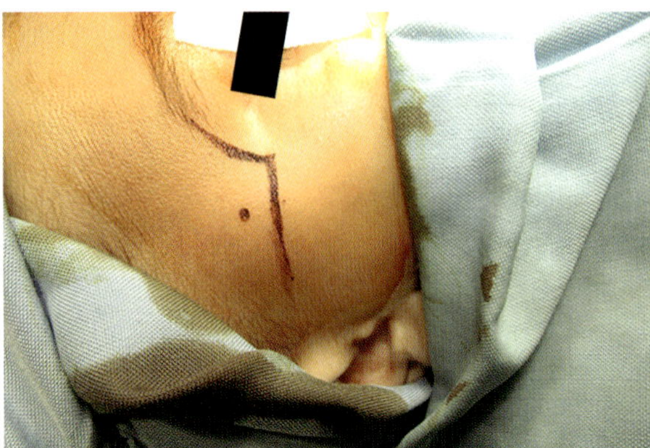

**Fig. 2.7:** Bilateral suprazygomatic maxillary nerve block : needle is passed horizontally above angle formed by posterior orbital margin and zygomatic arch. The direction of needle is change towards nasolabial fold after touching greater wing of sphenoid. The local anesthetic is injected in pterygopalatine fossa

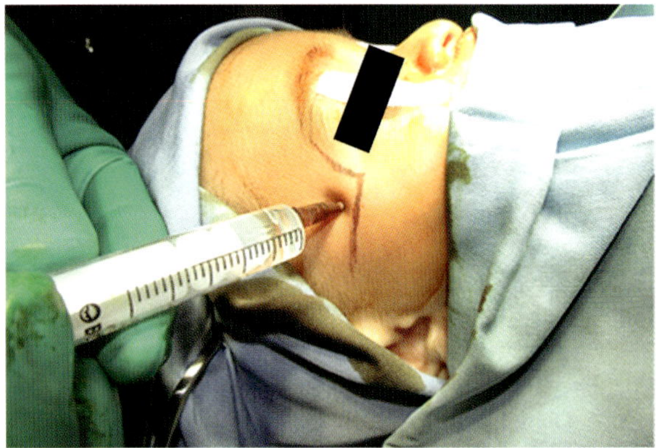

**Fig. 2.8:** Right suprazygomatic maxillary nerve block

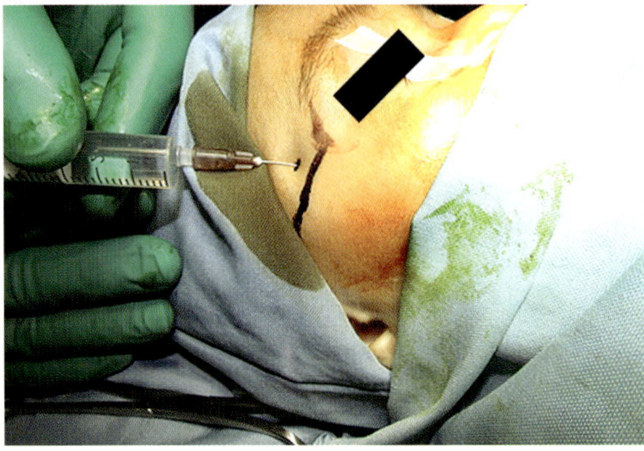

**Fig. 2.9:** Left suprazygomatic maxillary nerve block

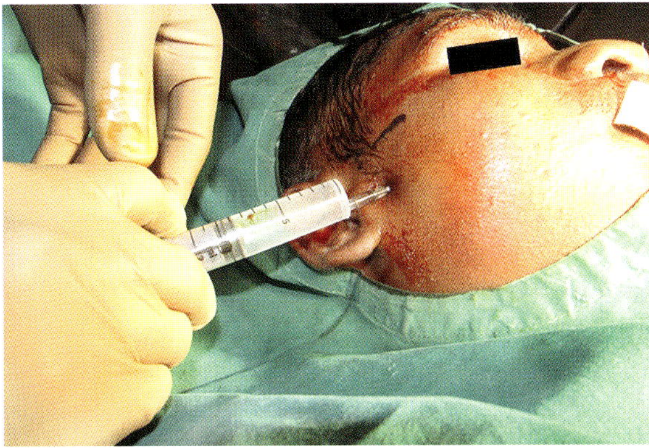

**Fig. 2.10:** Right infrazygomatic maxillary nerve block: Needle is passed below zygomatic arch and in front of mandibular condyle into infratemporal fossa

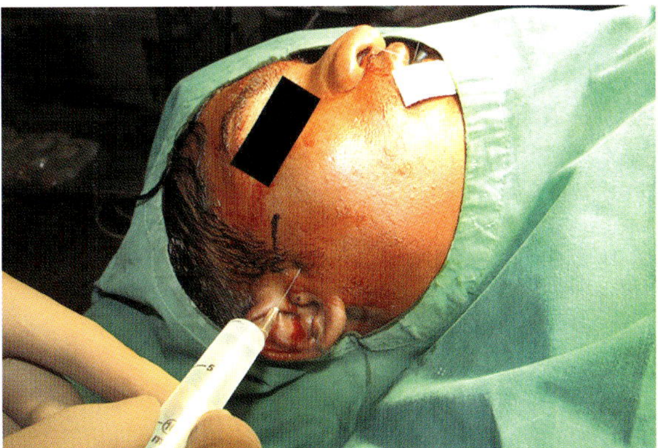

**Fig. 2.11:** Right infrazygomatic maxillary nerve block

reduces pain postoperative period. We use lignocain hydrochloride injection 2% 2.5 mg/kg and bupivacaine 0.5% 1 mg/kg dilute with water for injection in equal amount.[16]

## Bilateral Infrazygomatic Maxillary Nerve Block

Bilateral infrazygomatic maxillary nerve blocks[15,17] are more effective in adult patients. Needle is passed below zygomatic arch and in front of mandibular condyle in infratemporal fossa. Needle is directed forward so anesthetic solution will pass in pterygopalatine fossa through pterygomaxillary fissure.

## REFERENCES

1. Hatch DJ. Airway Management in cleft lip and palate surgery. Br J Anaesthesia. 1996;76:755-6.
2. Hnriksson Th, Skoog Vt. Identification of children at high anaesthetic risk at the time of primary palatoplasty. Scand J Plast Reconstr Surg Hand Surg. 2001;35:177-82.

3. Murat I, Constant I, Maud'huy M. Perioperative anaesthetic morbidities in children: a database of 24,165 anaesthetics over a 30-month period. Paediatr Anaesth. 2004;14;158-6.

4. Machotte A. Anaesthetic management of paediatric cleft lip and palate repair. Anaesthetist. 2005;54:455-66.

5. Muthukumar M, Arya VK, Mathew PJ, Sharma RK. Comparison of haemodynamic responses following different concentrations of adrenaline with or without lignocaine for surgical field infiltration during cleft lip and palate surgery in children. Anaesth Intensive Care. 2012;40:114-9.

6. Takemura H, Yasumoto K, Toi T, Hosoyawada A. Correlation of cleft type with incidence of perioprative respiratory complications in infants with cleft lip and palate. PAED Anaesthesia. 2002;12:585-8.

7. Trenlett M, Anaesthesia for cleft lip and palate surgery. Curr Anae Criticare. 2004;15:309-16.

8. Ugboko V, Olasoji Ho, Out yemi OD, Ogunbodede EO. The use of local anaesthesia in adult cleft lip repair: Case reports and review of the literature. Sahel Med J. 2001;4:135-7.

9. Jone RG. A short history of anaesthesia for hare lip and cleft palate repair. Br J Anaesth. 1971;43:796-802.

10. Law RC, de kler KC. Anaesthesia for cleft lip and palate surgery. Update in Anaeshesia. 2002;14(Article 9).

11. Biazon J, Peniche AC. Retrospective study of postoperative complications in primary lip and palate surgery. Rev Esc Enferm USP. 2008;42:519-25.

12. S Ahuja, Datta A, Krishna A, Bhattacharya A. Infraorbital nerve block for relief of postoperative pain following cleft lip surgery in infants. Anaesthesia. 1994;49:441-4.

13. Bosenberg AT, Kimble FW. Infraorbital nerve block in neonates for cleft lip repair. Anatomic study and clinical application. Br. J Anaesth.1995;74:506-8.

14. Gunawardana RH. Difficult laryngoscopy in cleft lip and palate surgery. Br J Anaesthesia. 1996;76:757-9.

15. Chiono J, Raux O, Bringuier S, Sola C, Bigorre M, Capdevila X, et al. Bilateral suprazygomatic maxillary nerve block for cleft palate repair in children: a prospective, randomised, double-blind study versus placebo. Anaesthesiology. 2014;120:1362-9.

16. Somerville N, Fenlon S. Anaesthesia for cleft lip and palate surgery. CEACCP. 2005;5:76-9.

17. Stajcic Z, Todorovic L. Blocks of the foramen rotandum and the oval foramen: a reappraisal of extraoral maxillary and mandibular nerve injections. Br J Oral Maxiloface Surg. 1997;35:328-33.

# CHAPTER 3

# Embryology

## CLASSICAL THEORY

Dursy (1869) and His (1874) postulated that there were five processes of the face, namely the frontonasal, the paired maxillary and mandibular processes. These processes grew towards and fused with each other, to form the face. Failure to fuse was thought to lead to cleft formation. This theory was too pat and did not serve to explain the formation of median clefts. Patten (1971) still believes that the theory of merging of process is essentially true and the mesoderm underneath gradually elevates the depressed lines of juncture.

## MESODERMAL REINFORCEMENT

Stark (1954) was stimulated in to a different line of thinking after reading about the work of Hochstetter (1936) who suggested that upper lip and premaxilla are represented by an epithelial wall into which reinforcing mesoderm must migrate to give substance to the lip (Fig. 3.1). This theory was first supported by Veau (1937) and Tondury (1955). Stark managed to six cleft embryos, three of which had bilateral clefts, and after serial coronal section and planimetric

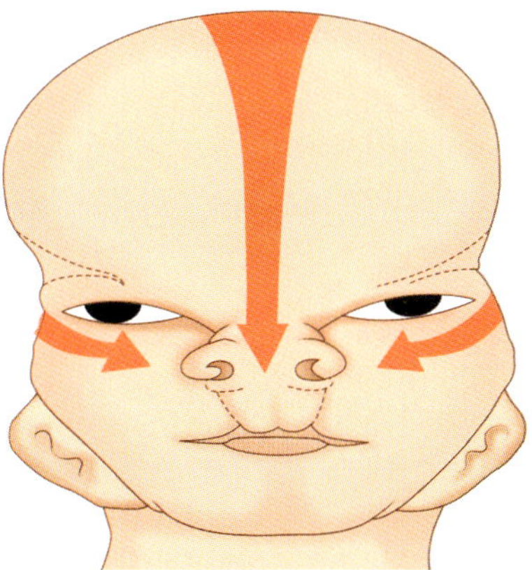

**Fig. 3.1:** Migration of mesoderm

measurements, he found of deficiency of mesoderm on the cleft side in every case and postulated his theory of mesodermal penetration.

His theory states that there are three mesodermal masses within that epithelial wall which constitutes the primitive palate. If mesoderm is deficient on one side, then the epithelial wall rupture on that is lacking, the cleft is either complete or incomplete . The Simonart's band which is present in incomplete cleft, was found to have only an epithelial cord of cells with no mesoderm. This served to emphasize the fact that this band was not a dynamic attempt at fusion of the cleft by a stream of mesoderm, as was previously thought, but rather, remnant of the epithelial wall which split up to the nostril, and stop short there.

Cranial neural crest cells give rise to most of the facial tissue including those forming the lip and palate. Much of the blueprint for the midfacial development is laid down very early at about 17th gestational day, in human embryos. Cranial neural crest cells migrate from their original position at the margins of the neural fold. At the most craniocaudal levels and in most specifies they migrate at the time of neural fold closer, either down beside the neural tube or laterally under the surface ectoderm. In the head region, crest cells migrating laterally and ventrally under the surface ectoderm are much more numerous and eventually differentiate in to all of the facial skeletal and connective tissues except the enamel of the teeth.

At the end of their migration crest cells form virtually all the mesenchyme in the upperfacial region, whereas in the visceral arches, the neural crest cells surround cores of mesodermal mesenchyme that were present before migration of endothelial linings of the embryonic blood vessels (Figs 3.2A to F).

The facial development enters a new phase at the end of 5th week of gestational age. It is manifested by the regional growth of visceral arches and facial prominences. A mesenchymal cell process meshwork is found in close contact with underside of epithelial areas. These mesenchymal cells connected by gap junction, mediate the epithelial mesenchymal interaction.

The olfactory placodes are epithelial thickenings, derived directly from the anterior margin in later development.

Initially, the olfactory placodes site over the corner of the forebrain so that its medial edge is more forward than its lateral edge. A curling forward of its lateral margin initiates formation of the lateral nasal process and causes it to grow further rapidly and "catch up" with the medial nasal process which forms at the medial edge and the placode.

The maxillary prominence is formed by the proximal half of first visceral arch, which bends so that its more proximal part end up facing forward under the eye. It then grows forward at its tip, which eventually contacts the medial nasal process and lateral nasal process.

As the morphogenetic movements continue, the lateral nasal process becomes progressively more developed and sweeps forward over the underlying maxillary prominence. The maxillary process has already made

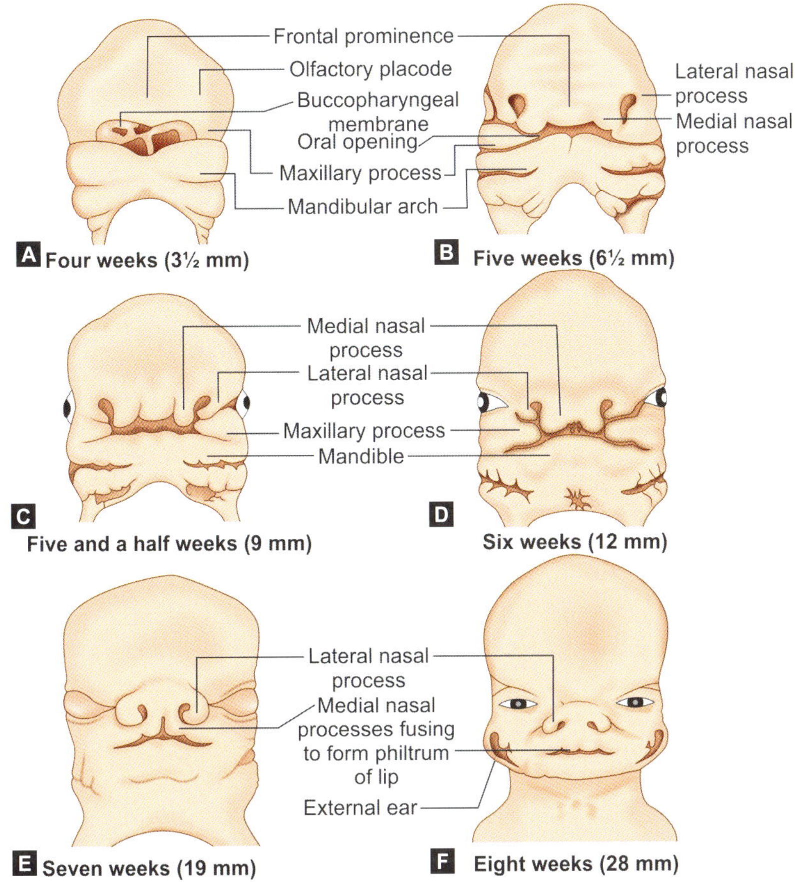



**Figs 3.2A to F:** Embryology. Normal development of face

contact with medial nasal process. With continue development, mostly growth in forward direction, lateral nasal process comes in contact with the medial nasal process. These prominences then coalesce through the phenomenon of fusion and margin.

Palatal process a plate like shelf grows medially from maxillary process. So, palate is formed by primitive palate, a part of frontonasal process and two palatal processes. Initially palatal shelves extend vertically and then rotate to a horizontal plane dorsal to the tongue.

Single mutation in multiple signaling pathway leads to multifactorial disorder facial cleft. There are three unique features in craniofacial development.

1. Dual origin of craniofacial tissue
   a. Cranial neural crest
   b. Mesoderm
2. Tissue interaction between neuroectoderm and facial ectoderm
3. Passive cell displacement and active cell migration, that defines head development.

The embryoblast grows and divides into three layers: ectoderm, mesoderm and endoderm. Embryo has cranial and caudal regions. Group of cells of primitive node forms primitive streak at caudal end of embryo. Craniocaudal and mediolateral axes are established. Sonic hedgehog helps subdivision of dumbbell-shaped area of future eye field (Figs 3.3A and B). Loss of shh in medial neural plate is responsible for cyclopia with proboscis. The neural plate rolls up to form neural tube to devide ectoderm in to neuroectoderm and non-neuroectoderm. Bone morphogenetic protein regulates growth in lateral crest cells emerges at junction of neural and non-neural ectoderm. Ephrin and Eph help neural crest cell migration.

TGF-B3 are important for fusion of palatal shelves. Defective in Wnt signaling leads to cleft formation due to insufficient growth of the maxillary prominence.

Forkhead box protein E1 (FOXE1) mutation supresses fusion between maxillary and nasal processes. Interferor regulatory factor (IRF6) deficit causes Van Der Woude syndrome and popliteal pterygium syndrome and isolated cleft lip and cleft palate.

Retinoic acid, a metabolite of vitamin A, in excess or in deficit can lead to microphthalmia, holoprosencephaly, cleft lip and cleft palate. Teratogenic dose of retinoic acid inhibits shh in frontonasal process epithelium.

Fetal alcohol syndrome, prenatal exposure to alcohol cause physical and mental impairement. Alcohol increases retinoic acid degradation and impairs retinoic acid synthesis. Ethanol disrupt hedgehog signaling activity leading to neural crest cell death and craniofacial defect.

Cyclopamine and jervine are active compound in *Veratrum californicum*. These steroidal alkaloids inhibit cholesterol synthesis and transport leading to cyclopia.

## ETIOLOGY

The embryological event occurs leading to cleft lip with or without cleft palate during 3–7 weeks and leading to cleft palate occurs during 5–12 weeks. The cleft

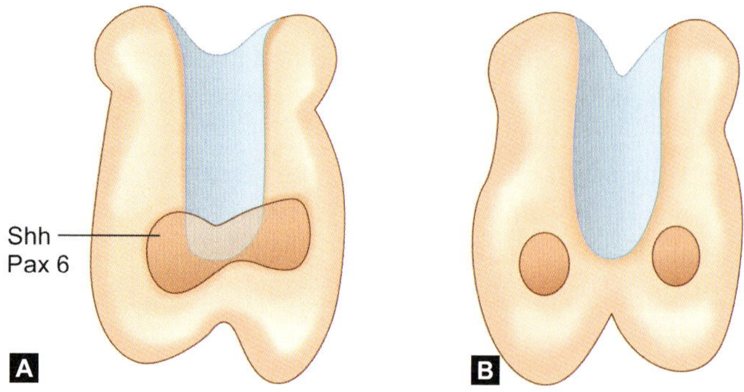


**Figs 3.3A and B:** Sonic hedgehog helps subdivision of dumbbell shaped area of future eye field

lip with or without palate in white American occurs one in 700–1000 babies. Boys are affected twice than girls. Cleft palate occurs 0.5 in 1000 population and girls are more affected than boys. Left unilateral cleft lip is more common than right unilateral cleft lip. Fogh-Andersen, 1942 noted distribution according to type of cleft of 25% cleft lip alone, 50% cleft lip and palate and 25% isolated cleft palate. Wilson, 1972 noted the unilateral left sided cleft lip right sided cleft lip and bilateral cleft lip occurs in a 6:3:1 relationship.

## Syndromic Cleft Lip with or without Cleft Palate

1. Trisomy 13 and trisomy 21
2. Waardenburg's syndrome
3. Van der Woude syndrome (Fig. 3.4)
4. Velocardiofacial syndrome
5. Stickler syndrome
6. Treacher-Collins syndrome
7. Downs syndrome
8. Goldenhar syndrome
9. Fetal alcohol syndrome

There are more than 200 syndromes associated with cleft lip and palate (Figs 3.5 to 3.10).

## Environmental Factors

1. Vitamin B deficiency
2. Vitamin A deficiency and vitamin A excess
3. Viral infection during first trimester
4. Exposure to radiation
5. Influence of drugs
   a. Cortisone
   b. Deoxyguanosine

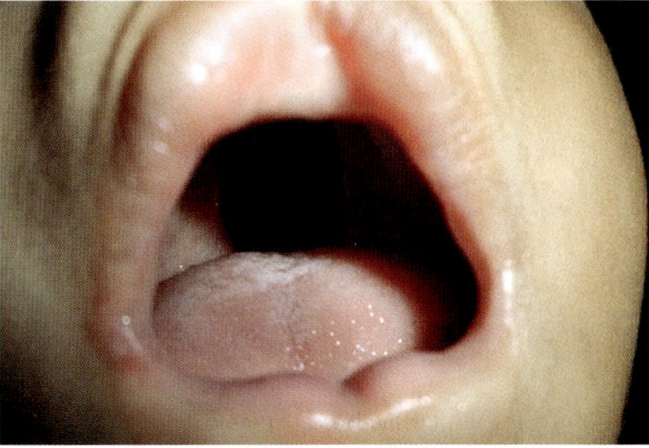

**Fig. 3.4:** Van der Woude syndrome

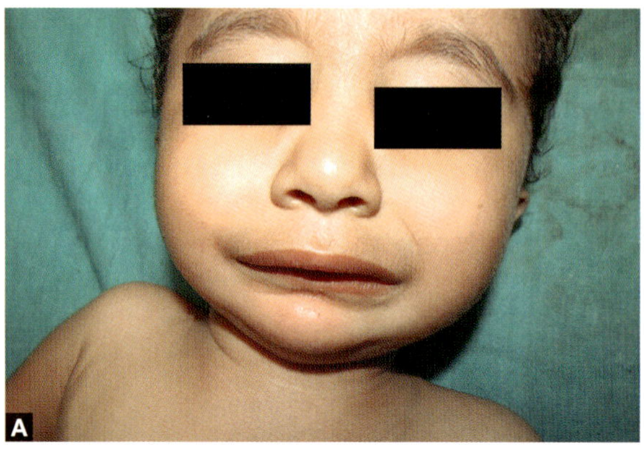

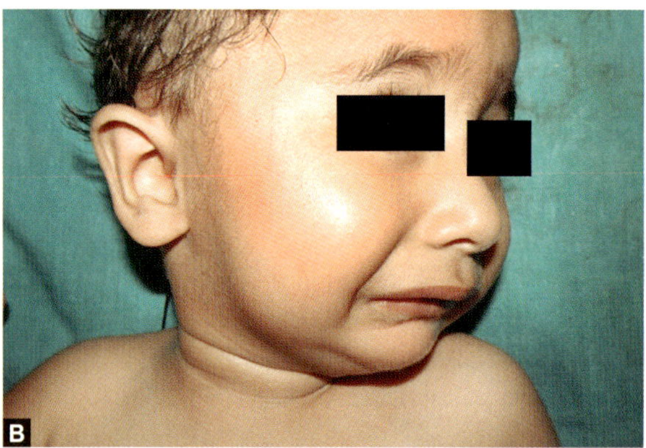

**Figs 3.5A and B:** Pierre-Robin sequence

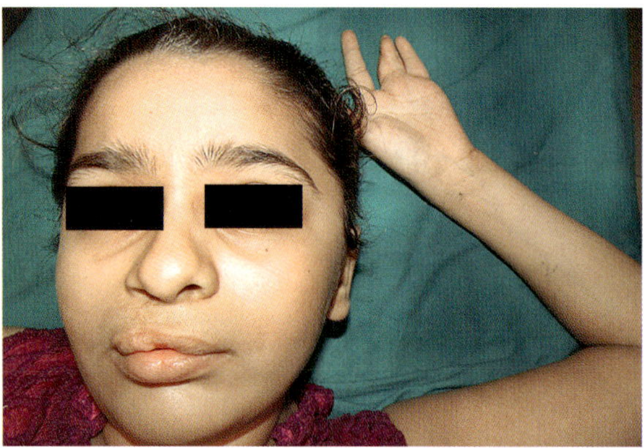

**Fig. 3.6:** Syndactyly: Right unilateral cleft lip

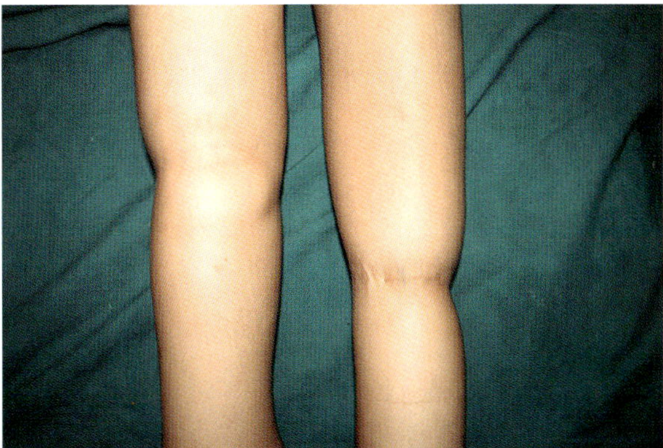

**Fig. 3.7:** Constriction ring syndrome

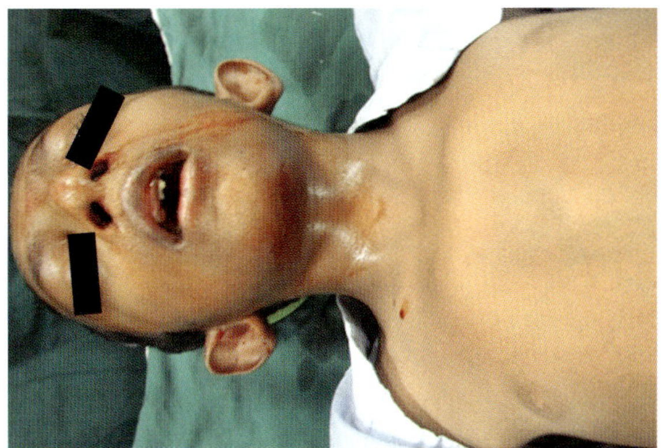

**Fig. 3.8:** Bilateral cleft lip and palate with chest wall deformity

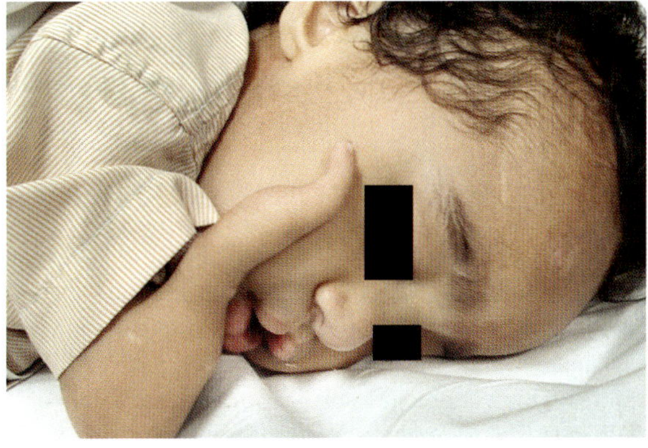

**Fig. 3.9:** Congenital deformity of right upper limb with bilateral cleft lip

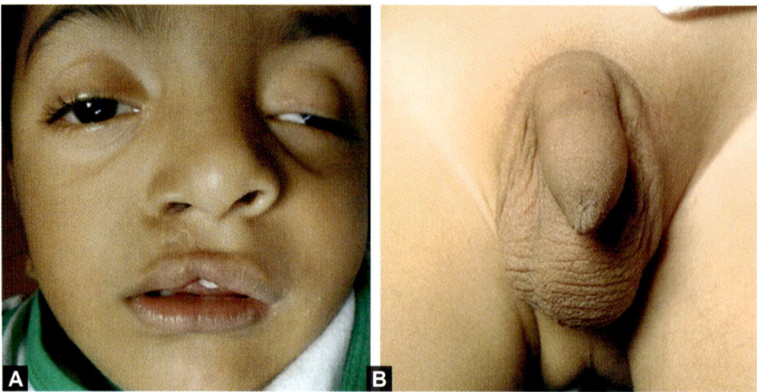

**Figs 3.10A and B:** (A) Right unilateral cleft lip with (B) Left congenital hydrocele

   c. Insulin
   d. Alcohol
   e. Cyclopamine
6. Anoxia
7. Stress
8. Smoking.

## BIBLIOGRAPHY


1. Ardinger HH, Buetow KH, Bell GI, et al. Association of genetic variation of the transforming growth factor—alpha gene with cleft lip and palate. Am J Huin Henet. 1989;45:348-53.
2. Chenevix-Trench G, Jones K, Green AC, et al. Cleft lip with or without cleft palate, associations with transforming growth factor alpha and retinoic acid receptor loci. An J hum Genet. 1992;51:1397-85.
3. Diewart VM, Shiota K. Morphology of human cleft lip embryos. Teratology. 1988;37:452.
4. Falconer DS. The inheritance of liability to certain diseases estimated from incidence among relatives. Ann Hum Genet. 1965;29:51.
5. Fraser FC. William allan memorial award Adress: evolution of a palatable multifactorial threshold model. Am J Hum Genet. 1980;32:796-813.
6. Fogh-Andersen P. Inheritance of harelip and cleft palate. Copenhagen: Nyt Nordisk Forlag. 1942.
7. Jones MC. Facial clefting. Etiology and developmental pathogenesis. Clin Plast Surg. 1993;20:599-606.
8. Lidral AC, Remitti PA, Basarat AM, et al. Association of MSx1 and TGFB3 with nonsyndromic clefting in humans. An J Hum Genet. 1998;63:557-68.
9. McKusick VA. Online Mendelian Inheritance in Man (OMIM). McKusick-Nathans Institute for Genetic Medicine, Johns Hopkins University (Baltimore, MD) and National Centre for Biotechnology Information, National library of Medicine, 2004.
10. Prescott NJ, Winter RM, Malcolm S. Nonsyndromic cleft lip and palate: complex genetics and environmental effects. Ann Hum Genet. 2001;65:505-15.

11. Rollnick BR, Pruzansky S. Genetic services at a centre for craniofacial anomalies. Cleft palate J. 1981;18:304-13.
12. Spritz RA. The genetics and epigenetics of orofacial clefts. Curr Opin Pediatr. 2001;13:556-60.
13. Tolarova. Periconceptional supplementation with vitamin and folic acid to prevent recurrence of cleft lip. Lancet. 1982;2:217.
14. Tondury G. On the mechanism of cleft formation. In: Pruzansky S, (Ed). International symposium on congenital anomalies of the face and associated structures (Charles C Thomas: Springfield 1961). 85-101.
15. Wyszynki DF, Maestry N, McIntosh I, et al. Evidence for an association between markers on chromosome 199 and nonsyndromic cleft lip with or without cleft palate in two groups of multiplex families. Hum Genet. 1997;99:22-26.

# CHAPTER 4

# Anatomy

The lips form the first part of alimentary canal. It is more observed and known for its beauty color and shape rather than the fact that it is the entrance to a life support system.

The lips are two fleshy folds which surround the oral orifice. The upper lip is attached above to the nose and blends laterally in to the lower lip at the commisures. The upper lip protrudes a little in relation to the lower lip in the normal individual. Columella stands as a graceful central column, straight and narrow, right up to the nasal tip. The arches of alae are symmetrical, with equal bulges of the alar cartilage in the nasal tip (Fig. 4.1).

The ideal length of the upper lip at rest, places its inferior edge at the lower one third of the upper incisor teeth. As the upper lip rises, the more of the incisors are revealed until with similing, there is three fourth incisor exposure.

The mucocutaneous junction of the upper lip is an uninterrupted 1–2 mm rounded roll from commisure to commisure which tops the vermilion and pick up white light. It coincides in its curves with undulation of the cupid's bow of the vermilion which has a central free border tubercle flanked by a slight

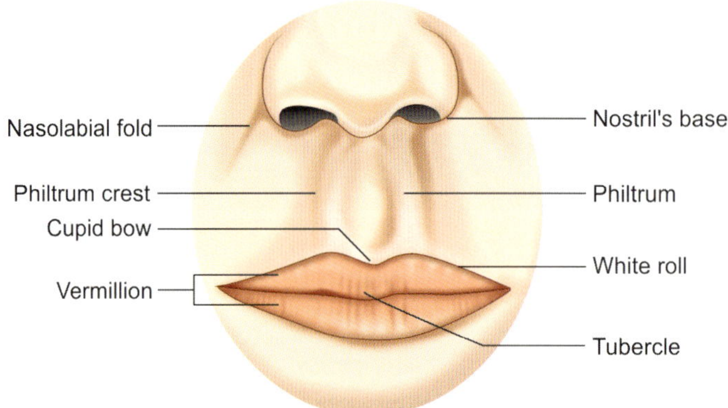


**Fig. 4.1:** Anatomy

indentation. From the height of each arch of the bow, the philtral columns curve upward toward the base of columella. Between these columns is philtrum hollow or dimple which accentuates the effect of the eminence.

The vermilion is transitional zone in which the epithelium is thin and non-keratinized. The connective tissue papillae are numerous, densely arranged, slender and extend close to the surface epithelial cell layers. The abundance of eleidin in the epithelial cell layers, increases translucency while numerous rich capillaries of the papillae, create the red color of this area.

The mucous membrane on the deeper aspect is lighter in color, when compared with the vermilion.

## ORBICULARIS ORIS MUSCLE[1,2]

Charpy and Poirier (1904) and lightoller (1925) published its normal anatomy. It is the principle muscle of the lip and passes partially around the entire oral fissure. It is in intimate contact anteriorly with the skin and posteriorly with mucous membrane. It consists anatomically and functionally of the two parts, the superficial and deep (Figs 4.2 and 4.3).

In the upper lip, these fibers decussate in the midline to insert in to the opposite philtral column.[3,4] The study of philtrum by Latham and Deaton (1976) confirmed the same.[3] It also demonstrated that the philtral column, in addition to orbicularis oris contains fibers of levator labii superiors in lower parts and nasalis in upper part. The muscle of facial expression intermingles with orbicularis oris and participates in its function by their dilating or stabilizing effect or both.

The superficial portion of the muscle brings the lips together.[5,6] Each fibers also contact independently to provide fine shades of expression. The deep layers of muscle encircle the orifice of mouth and function solely as constrictor of mouth.

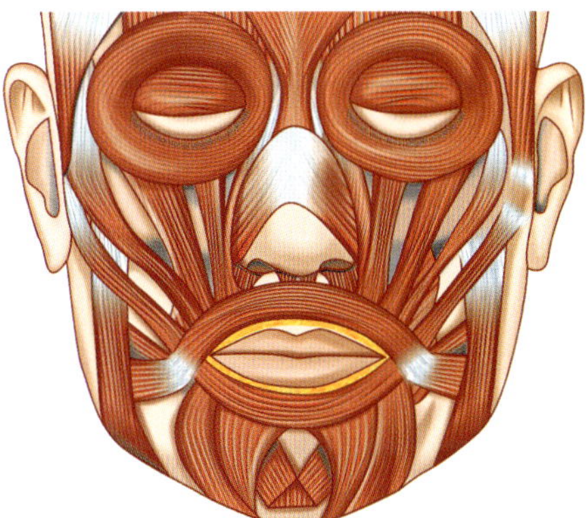

**Fig. 4.2:** Orbicularis oris muscle[2]

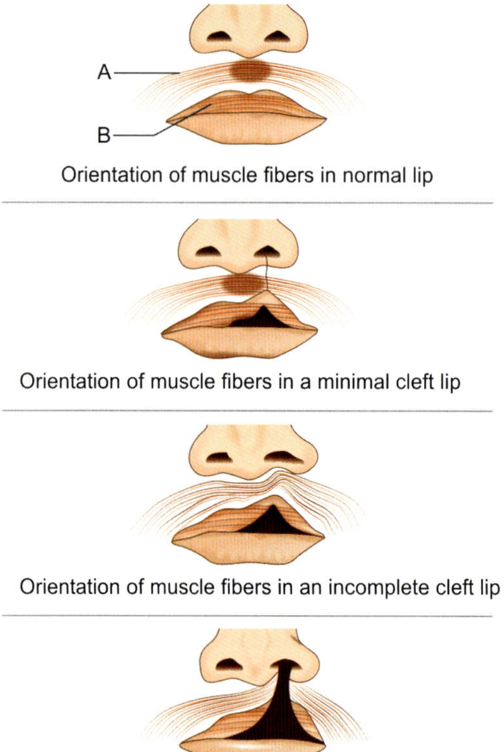



**Fig. 4.3:** Orientation of muscle fibers in upper lip

## CLEFT MUSCLES IN UNILATERAL CLEFT LIP[7,8]

### Complete Unilateral Cleft Lip

- Complete unilateral orbicularis oris muscle do not decussate transversely across the midline. They proceed horizontally from the commissure towards the midline, then turn upward along the margins of the cleft laterally beneath the base of the alae of the nose and medially beneath the base of the columella. Here, most of the fibers attach to the periosteum of the maxilla while a few disappear in subcutis.

### Incomplete Unilateral Cleft Lip

1. Major incomplete unilateral cleft lip: In this, only narrow bridge is formed, and the arrangement of orbicularis oris muscle is similar to one seen in complete unilateral cleft lip.
2. Minor incomplete unilateral cleft lip: In this, the cleft does not exceed two-third of lip height and the muscle fibers reaches over the lip of the cleft and passes from lateral to medial lip segments. The muscle within the cleft, is intersespersed by the trabeculae of the collaginous connective

tissue. The musculature on the medial side is underdeveloped and does not extend as far forwards to the edge of the cleft as it does on the lateral side. These fibers, on lateral side, form a lump on contraction.

M Fara (1968) studied cleft lip in stillborn children by histological section and arteriogram and reported similar findings. He also stated that muscle fibers were absent in bridges of less than one-third height of the lip.

Kernahan (1978) studied anatomy of orbicularis oris muscle by electrical stimulation. He concluded that, on medial side, the fibers were scarce and ran transversely, and on lateral side, they were more abundant and insert in to dermis.

## Blood Supply

The main blood supply to the lip and nose area comes from the facial branch of the external carotid artery. The facial artery gives off inferior and superior labial arteries which arise near the corner of the mouth and course as close to the mucous membrane. The terminal branches of internal carotid artery and infraorbital artery also contribute to some extent (Fig. 4.4).

The lateral element of the cleft lip is supplied by the superior labial artery which follows the course of the orbicularis oris muscle bundles and courses upwards to the nasal ala, where it anastomoses with lateral nasal or angular artery. In incomplete clefts, the artery passes through bridges in the form of a thin terminal branch. On the medial element of the cleft, the course of the artery is similar but its diameter is visible smaller and its branches are fewer than lateral element into columella, where they anastomose mainly with posterior septal arteries.

## ANATOMY OF UNILATERAL CLEFT LIP AND NOSE

The typical nasal deformity associated with congenital unilateral cleft lip represents both discrepancy and a displacement of parts. It persists without

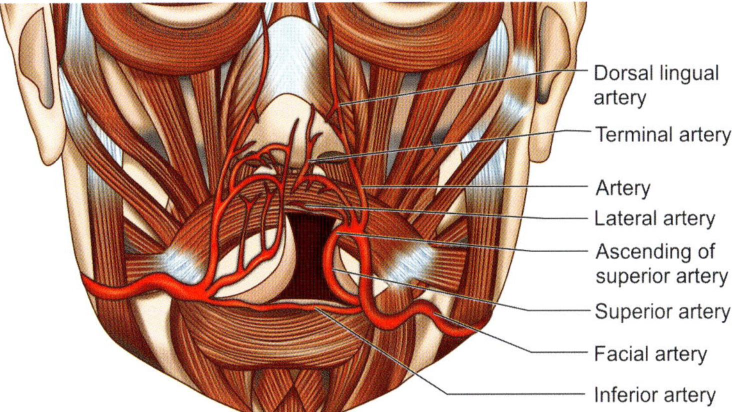


**Fig. 4.4** Blood supply of cleft lip

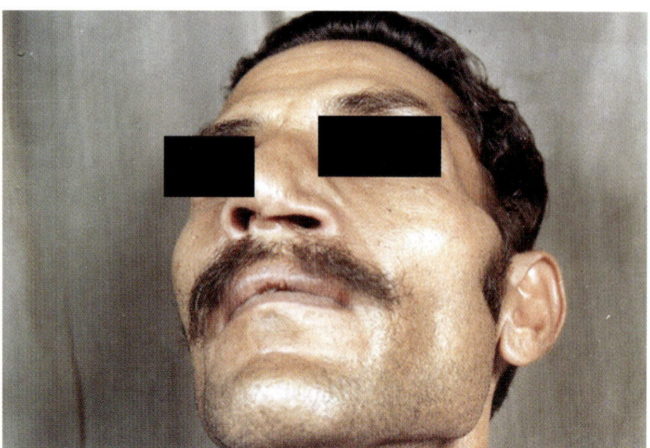

**Fig. 4.5:** Cleft nose

great improvement during growth. The distortion is confined to the cleft side only and is emphasized by comparison with normal opposite side (Fig. 4.5).

## Plateform

The actual plateform of the nose is cleft. This results in projection and outward rotation of the premaxilla and the retroposition of the lateral maxillary element.

## Septum

The medial maxillary element is forward and lateral maxillary segment is backward. This results in the twist and slant of the septum. The anterior portion of the septum tilts over the cleft. Its inferior edge may be dislocated out of the vomerine groove and present with the nasal spine in the floor of the normal nostril. This dislocation gives a twist to the nasal tip.

## Nasal Bones

The asymmetry of maxilla and premaxilla and the deviation of septum result in some distortions of the nasal bones.

## Columella

It is deflected by the deviation of the septum behind it. There is unilateral shortness in the vertical height on the side of the cleft. This can vary from the three fourth to two third to even on half that of normal side.

## Nasal Floor

In complete cleft, nasal floor is cleft not only in skin and muscle but also in bone. The position of the maxillary elements can vary from overlap to abutment to gaps of millimeters to centimeters. In incomplete clefts, there can be a variation from thin skin bridge across a very wide nasal floor within a millimeter of normal width.

## Lower Lateral Alar Cartilage

The alar cartilage on the cleft side are attenuated, the deformed alar cartilage on the cleft side is dislodged from its rightful balanced position besides its mate in the dome of the tip. Its medial crus are lower in the columella with the junction curve of the medial and lateral crus seperated from the opposite alar cartilage and resting below it. It is flattened and stretched across the cleft at an obtuse angle.

## Alar Crease

The alar crease on the normal side runs parallel to the upperborder of the lower lateral cartilage. It smoothes out as it approaches the bulge of the alar cartilage in the dome of the nasal tip. On the cleft side, the alar crease has no alar cartilage bulge to give way. Consequently, unopposed by this structure, it continues obliquely across the lip.

## Alar Base

The alar base is invariably rotated outwards producing a flare. It can be wider in bulk than normal or grooved.

## Alar Rim

There is skin cover without cartilage which droops over the alar rim like a web. This reduces the apparent length of the columella, on the cleft side.

## Vestibular Lining

The lining of the nasal vestibule seems to be stretched over a greater area, than on normal side, with actual eversion of lining in the alar base region.

## REFERENCES


1. De Mey A, Van Hoof I, De Roy G, Lejour M. Anatomy of the orbicularis oris muscle in cleft lip. Br J Plast Surg. 1989;6:710-4.
2. Dado DV, Kernahan DA. Anatomy of the orbicularis oris muscle in incomplete unilateral cleft lip based on histological examination. Ann Plast Surg. 1985;15:90-8.
3. Latham RA, Deaton TG. The structural basis of the philtrum and contour of the Vermilion border: a study of musculature of upper lip. J Anat. 1976;121:151.
4. Mulliken JB, Pensler JM, Kozake HP. The anatomy of cupid's bow in normal and cleft lip. Plast Reconstr Surg. 1993;92:395-404.
5. Mooney MP, Siegel MI, Kimes KR, Todhunter J. Development of the orbicularis oris muscle in normal and cleft lip and palate human fetuses using three-dimensional computer reconstruction. Plast Reconster Surg. 1988;81(3):336-45.

6. Schendel SA, Pearl RM, De'Armond SJ. Pathophysiology of cleft lip muscle. Plast Reconstr Surg. 1989;83(5):777-84.
7. Huarg MH, Lee ST, Rajendran K. A fresh cadaveric study of the paratubal muscle: implications for Eustachian tube function in cleft palate Plast. Reconstr Surg. 1997;100:833-42.
8. Kernahan DA, Dado DD, Bauer SB. The anatomy of orbicualaris oris muscle in unilateral cleft lip based on a three dimensional histologic reconstruction. Plast Reconstr Surg. 1989;73:875.

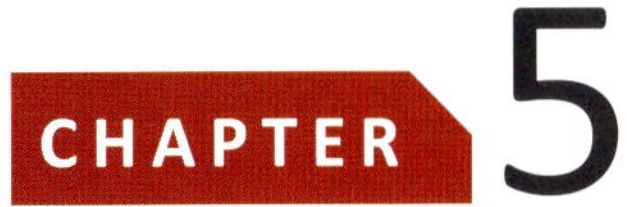

# CHAPTER 5

# Classification

Various classification systems[1-5] have been proposed, but only a few of the following have been found wide clinical acceptance.

## DAVIS AND RITCHIE (1922)[1]

Congenital clefts were divided into three groups according to the position to the alveolar process.

**Group 1:** Prealveolar clefts:
Unilateral, median or bilateral.

**Group 2:** Postalveolar clefts involving the soft palate only, the soft and hard palates or a submucous cleft palate.

**Group 3:** Alveolar clefts:
Unilateral, median or bilateral (Fig. 5.1).

## VEAU (1931)

Suggested a classification dividing patients into four groups:

**Group 1:** Cleft of soft palate only.

**Group 2:** Cleft of hard and soft palate extending no further than the incisive foramen thus,the secondary palate only.

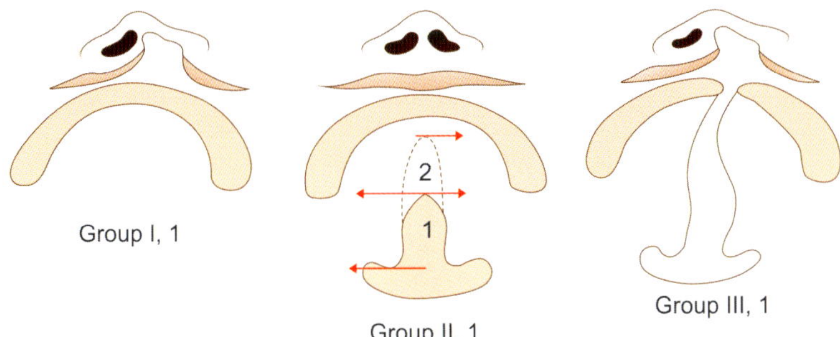



**Fig. 5.1:** Davis and Ritchie's classification

**Group 3:** Complete unilateral cleft extending from the uvuala to incisive foramen in the midline, then deviating to the one side and usually extending through the alveolus at the position of the future lateral incisor teeth.

**Group 4:** Complete bilateral cleft resembling group 3, with two clefts extending forward from the incisive foramen through the alveolus.

## KERNAHAN AND STARK (1958)

Proposed the need for a classification based on embryology rather than morphology.

## KERNAHAN (1971)[2]

Proposed a striped Y classification. The incisive foramen is the reference point. With stippling of the involved portion of the Y, the system provides rapid graphic presentation of the original pathological condition and leads itself to computer graphic presentation.

The right and left limbs of Y are divided in to three sections:

**The upper portion:** Lip 1 and 4

**The middle portion:** Alveolus 2 and 5

**The lower portion:** The hard palate from the alveolus to incisive foramen 3 and 6

The vertical limb is divided to three segments:

**Upper two segments:** Hard palate (7 and 8)

**Lower one segment:** Soft palate (9) (Fig. 5.2).

## MILLARD

Modified this stripped Y classification by adding inverted triangles over the apex of the Elsahy's triangular peaks to indicate nasal deformities. The triangular peak represents the nasal floor (Figs 5.3 to 5.17).

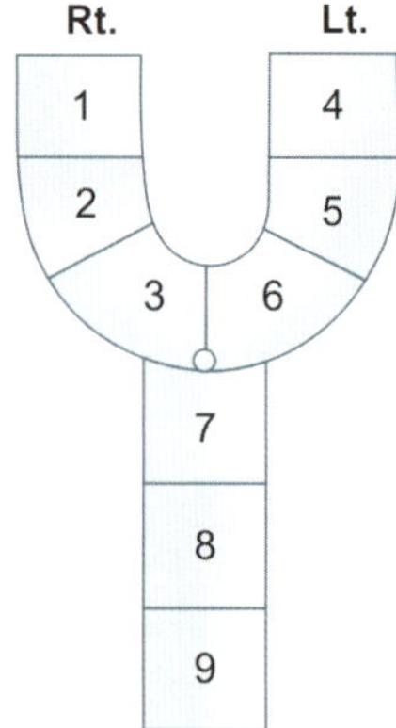


**Fig. 5.2:** Kernahan's Y symbolic classification

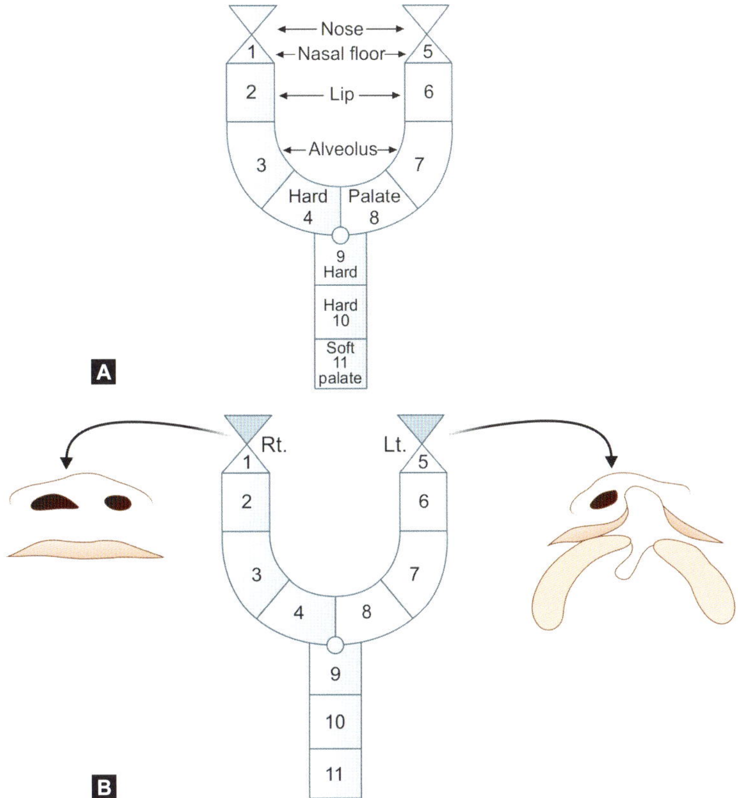



**Figs 5.3A and B:** Millard's modified stripped Y classification

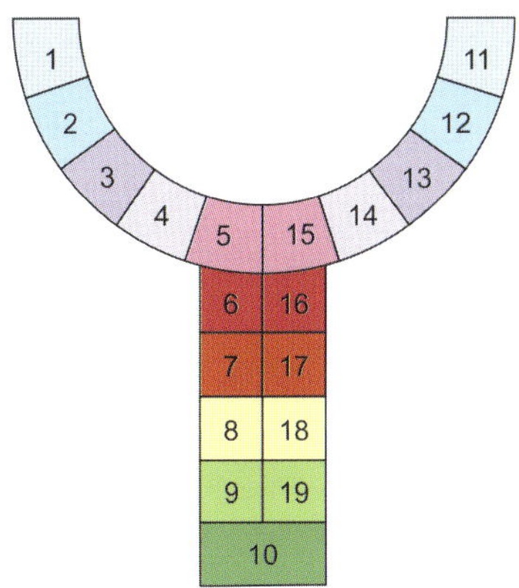



**Fig. 5.4:** Double Y classification of clefts

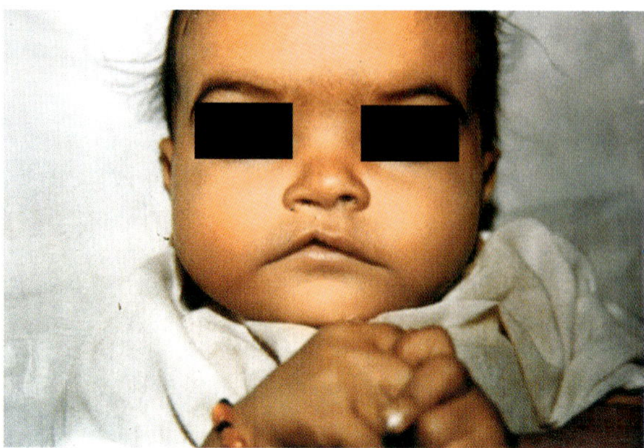

**Fig. 5.5:** Right microform cleft lip

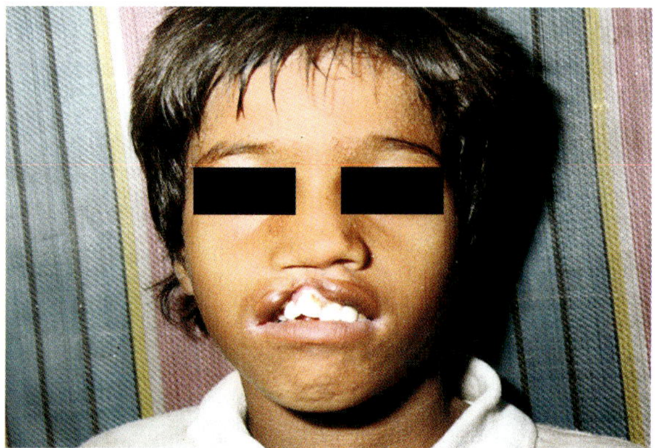

**Fig. 5.6:** Right incomplete cleft lip

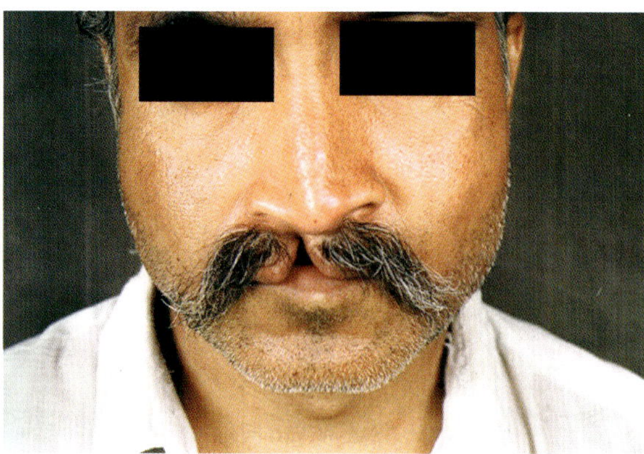

**Fig. 5.7:** Right complete cleft lip with normal alveolus (incomplete cleft of primary palate)

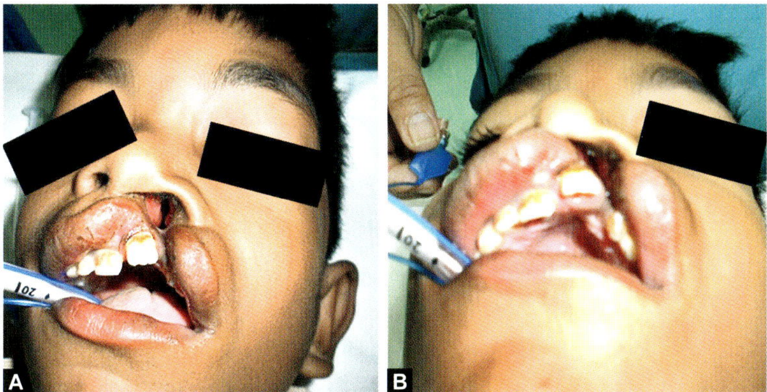

**Figs 5.8A and B:** Left complete cleft lip with cleft alveolus (complete cleft of primary palate left side)

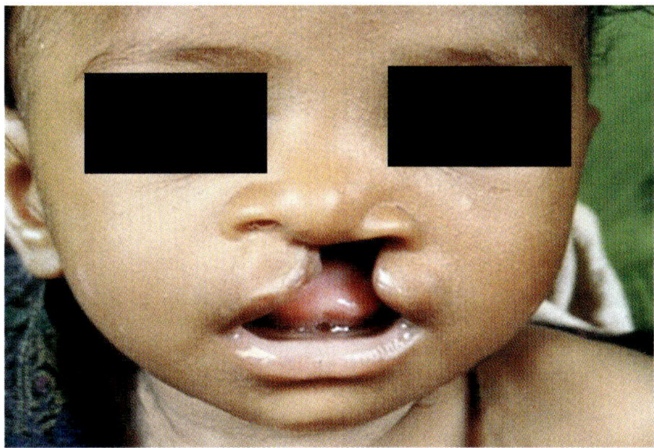

**Fig. 5.9:** Left complete cleft lip with palate

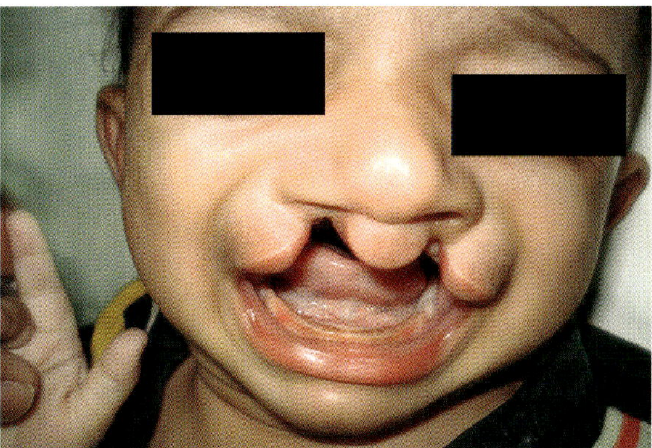

**Fig. 5.10:** Bilateral left lip

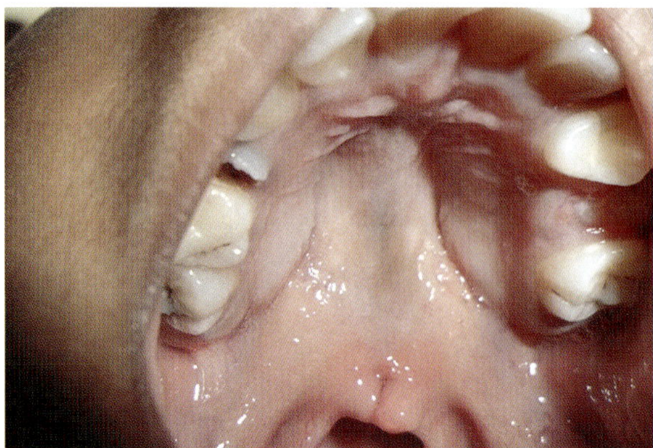

**Fig. 5.11:** Submucous cleft palate

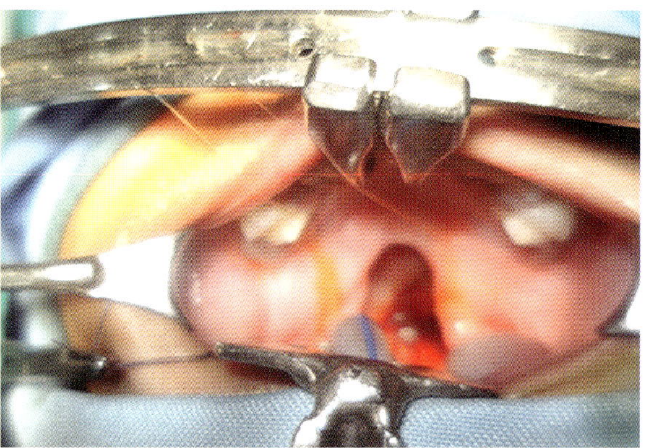

**Fig. 5.12:** Incomplete cleft palate

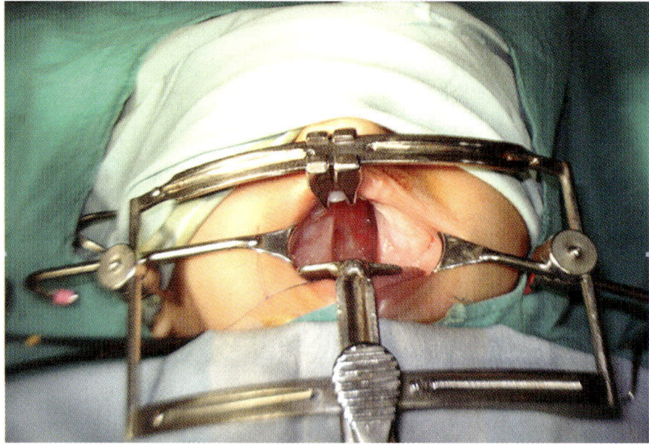

**Fig. 5.13:** Left cleft lip with palate

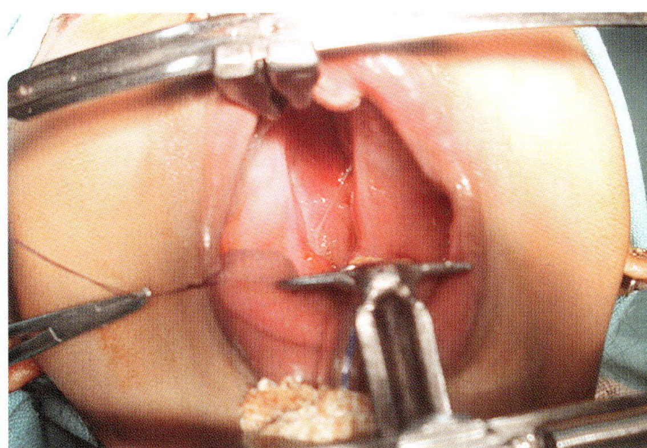

**Fig. 5.14:** Bilateral cleft lip with palate

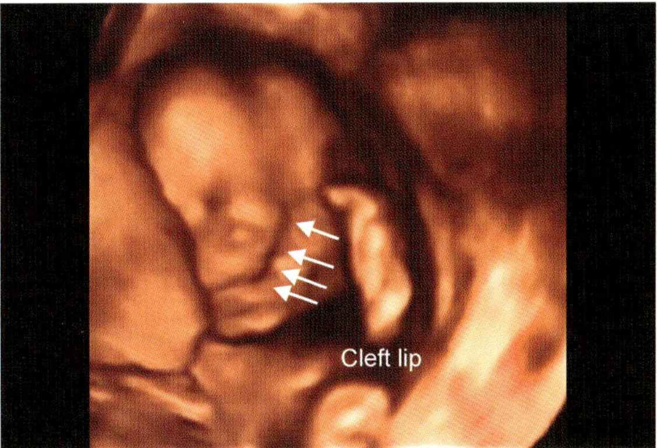



**Fig. 5.15:** 3D sonography during pregnancy showing left unilateral cleft lip

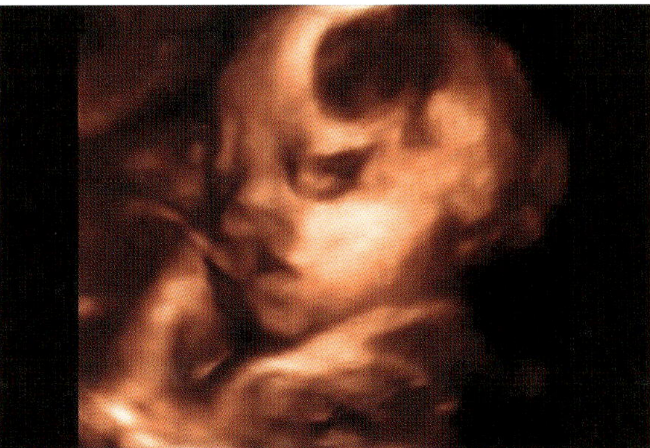

**Fig. 5.16:** 3D sonography showing left unilateral cleft lip

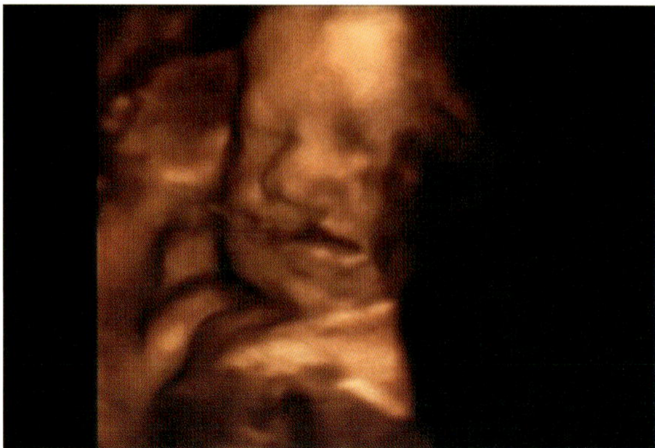

**Fig. 5.17:** One more view of the same patient

## HARKINS AND ASSOCIATES (1962)[3]

Presented pictorial classification based on the same embryological principles used by Kernahan and Stark.

## SPINA (1974)

Modified and simplified the Harkins classification.
Professor C. Balakrishnan devised a system of classification which can be used for computerized data processing.[4]
Cleft patients are classified by letter codes, R for right and L for left unilateral cleft lip. Second letter P for primary palate and S for secondary palate. Third letter I for incomplete and C for complete lesions.

## REFERENCES


1. Davis JS, Ritchie HP. Classification of congenital clefts of the lip and palate. JAMA. 1922;79:1323-7.
2. Kernahan DA, Stark RB. A new classification for cleft lip and cleft palate. Plast Reconstr Surg Transplant Bull. 1958;22(5):435-41.
3. Harkins CS, Berlin A. Harding RL. Longacre JJ, Snodgrasse RM. A classification of cleft lip and cleft palate. Plast Reconstr Surg. 1962;29:31-9.
4. Bakrishnan C. Indian classification of cleft lip and palate. Ind J Plast Surg. 1975;8(1):43-4.
5. Vilar-Sancho B. A proposed new international classification of congenital cleft lip and cleft palate. Plast Reconstr Surg Transplant Bull. 1962;30:263-6.

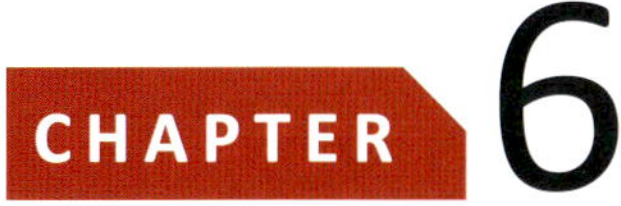

# Unilateral Cleft Lip Repair

PROFORMA

Name:                                    Date of Birth:

Age:                                     Parent's Age:

Sex:

Caste:

Address:

Date of Admission:

History:

- History of failure to thrive
- History of nasal regurgitation
- History of discharge from ear
- Cough, fever, dyspnea
- Difficulty in speech in children
- Family history
- Drugs taken during pregnancy
- Epilepsy in mother
- Radiation exposure during pregnancy
- Congenital deformities in family

## CLINICAL EXAMINATION

- Cleft lip[1]
- Cleft palate
- Side
- Extent
- Nasal deformities
- Middle ear
- Other congenital anomalies
- Respiratory tract and chest

## INVESTIGATION

Routine investigation like hemogram, urine examination, X-ray chest, cardiac status (whenever needed).

## TREATMENT

- Patients were operated after age of 3 months
- Weight should be more than 4 kg
- Hemoglobin percentage should be more than 10 g.

## PREOPERATIVE PREPARATION

We have admitted all patients one or two days prior to operation. The skin, nose, throat, teeth, ears, and chest are examined to ensure freedom from infection. Antibiotics were started one day prior to operation. Full feed was given six hours and plain fluid four hours before operation.

In adult patients preoperative measures consists of clipping of nasal hairs, cleaning of mouth and teeth and cleaning of face with soap. In male patients shaving of moustaches was carried out.

### Anesthesia

All patients were operated under general anesthesia with endotracheal intubation and throat pack.
- Preoperative evaluation
- History
  - Complaint of cough, running nose, fever in last 10 days
  - Any hospitalization for any major illness
  - Mother obstetric history
  - Immunization of child.
- Clinical examination
  - Respiratory any rhonchi and creps for chest infection
  - Cardiovascular system any congenital anomaly—murmur
  - General examination—any anomaly that correlate with any syndrome.

### Operation: Unilateral Cleft Lip Repair[2-25]

Unilateral cleft is one of the congenital malformations. In addition to facial disfigurement, patients with this type of malformation find their disability compounded by an inability to communicate with other in a satisfactory manner because when associated with cleft palate, there is difficulty in speech.

### Robert F Hegarty, Popularized His Triangular Flap Method in 1958[26]

In their outstanding contribution to cleft lip repair in 1930, Blair and Brown stated the logic of the Mirault plan was that a flap was taken from the upper part of the lip where there was excess tissue and implanted in the lower border where tissue was most needed.

In order to take even further advantage of the opportunities afforded by this basic concept Hegarty decided to preserve more tissue on the lateral side by the cleft and introduce it, into a notch created medially by drooping the cleft side of the cupid bow to its normal position.

By introducing tissue in this manner into the lower third of the lip, a more normal pout is obtained, notching of the lip is prevented, and tension on the suture line is reduced.

In essence, the cupid's bow on the cleft side of the midline is the dropped to the normal position and V-shaped defect, so created is filled with a flap of the proper dimension taken from the upper lateral side of the cleft. So as to utilize tissue this might be sacrificed in other procedures. In this manner are possible useful tissue is incorporated to avoid the undesirable effects and appearance of the tight lip (Figs 6.1 to 6.30).

## Robert F Hegarty's Triangular Flap Method[26]

This repair is reliable operation for a single cleft from the most incomplete to the very wide clefts.

A lip adhesion is not necessary as a preliminary operation before the definitive repair.

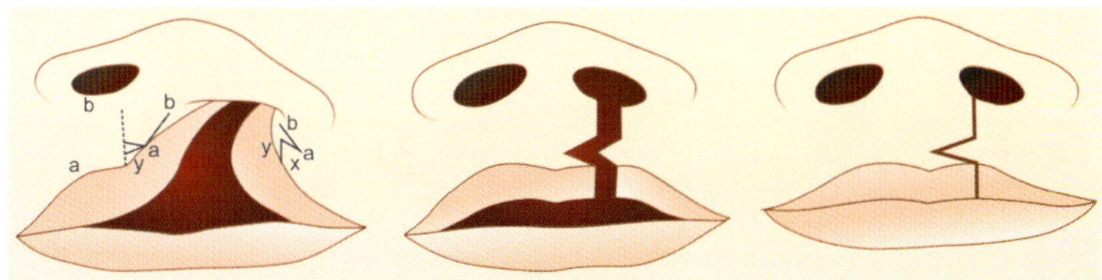

**Fig. 6.1:** Hegarty (1958) unilateral cleft lip repair

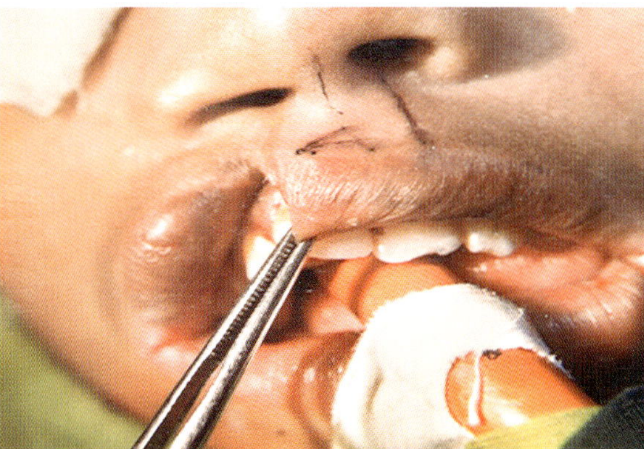

**Fig. 6.2:** Right incomplete unilateral cleft lip

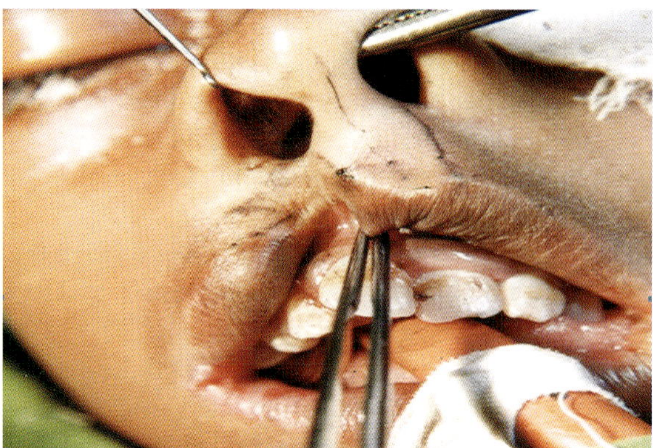

**Fig. 6.3:** Markings done

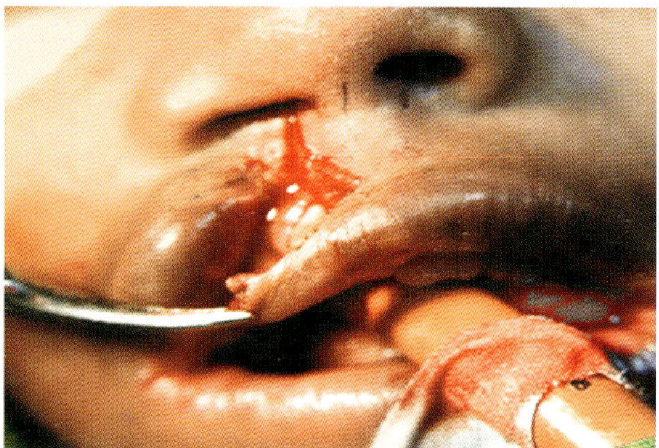

**Fig. 6.4:** Incision taken in medial side

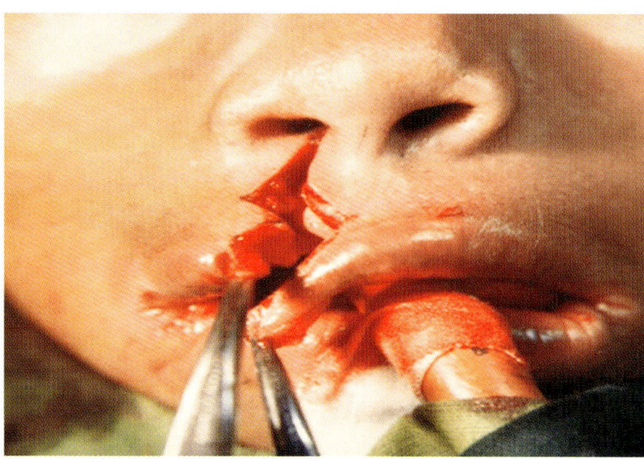

**Fig. 6.5:** Incision and dissection completed

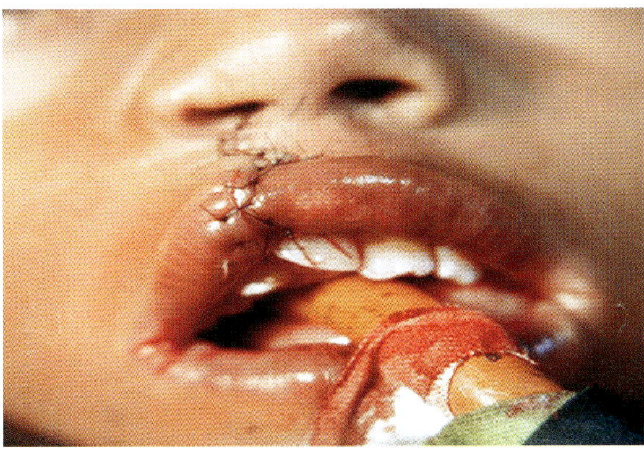

**Fig. 6.6:** Suturing completed

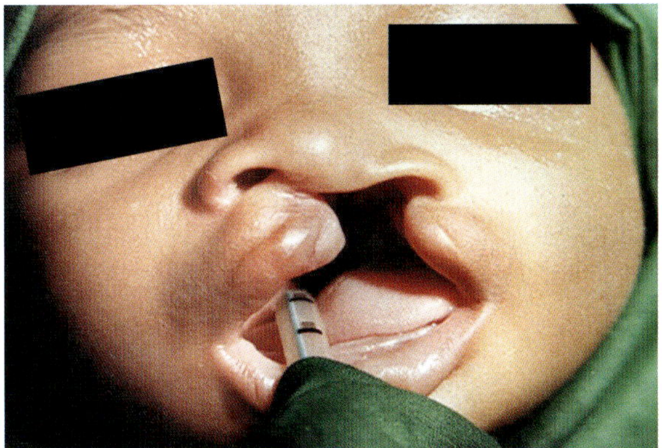

**Fig. 6.7:** Left unilateral cleft lip with palate

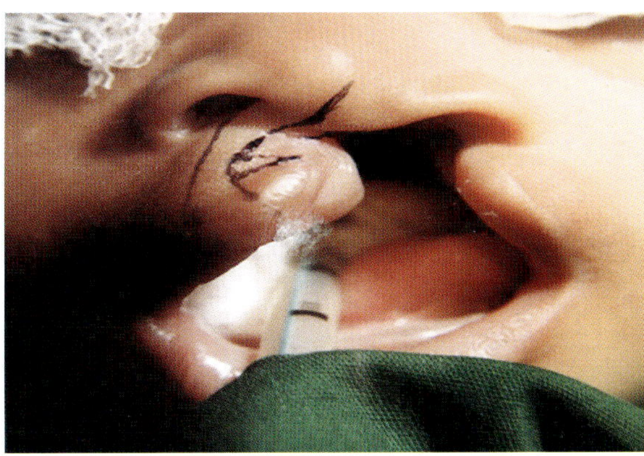

**Fig. 6.8:** Markings done medial side

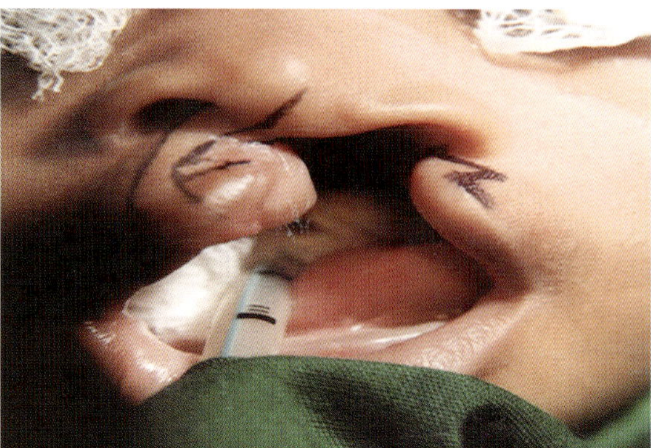

**Fig. 6.9:** Markings on lateral segment

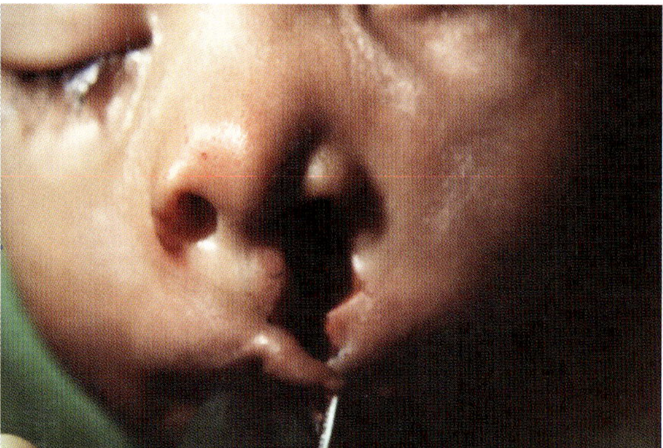

**Fig. 6.10:** Dissection completed

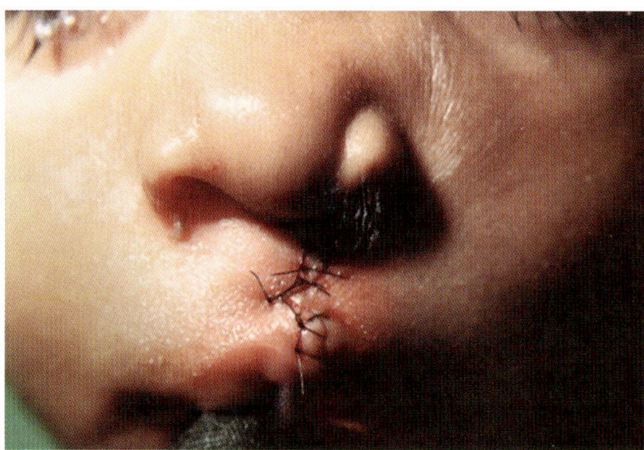

**Fig. 6.11:** Suturing completed 4-0 vicryl was used for muscle and mucosal repair and nylon 6-0 used for skin closure

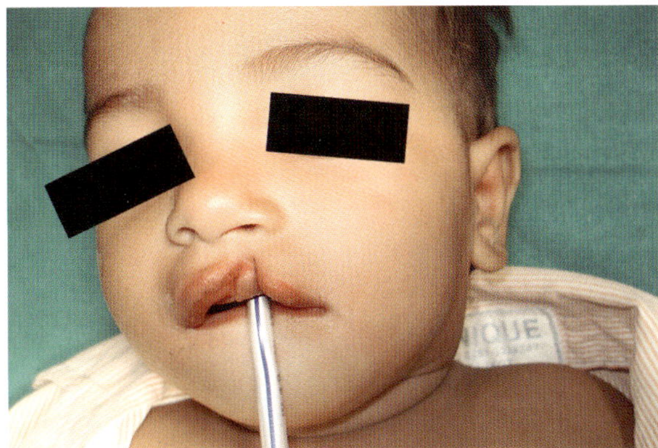

**Fig. 6.12:** Left incomplete unilateral cleft lip

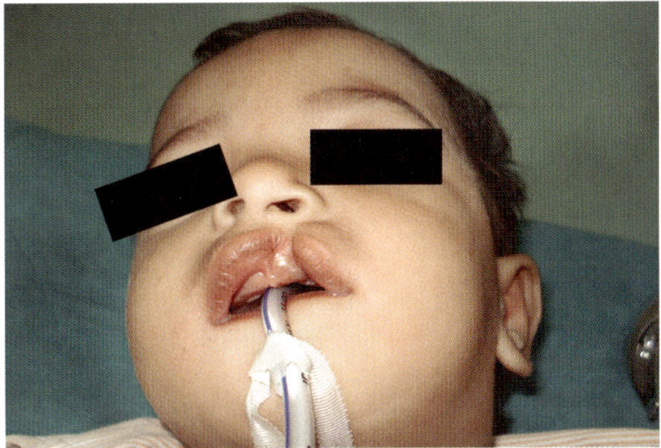

**Fig. 6.13:** Worms view of patient with left unilateral cleft lip

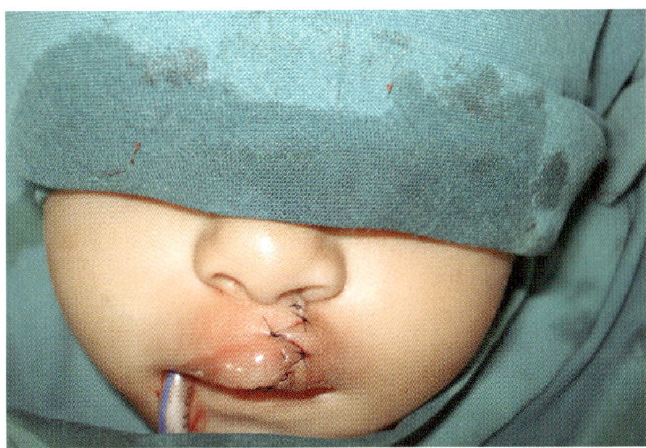

**Fig. 6.14:** Frontal view of repaired left unilateral cleft lip

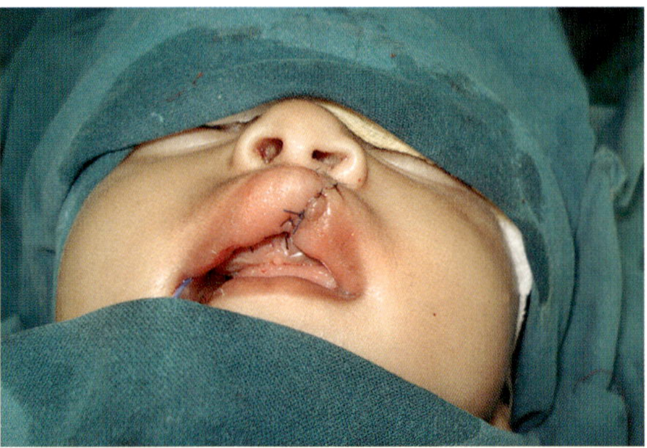

**Fig. 6.15:** Worms view of repaired left unilateral cleft lip

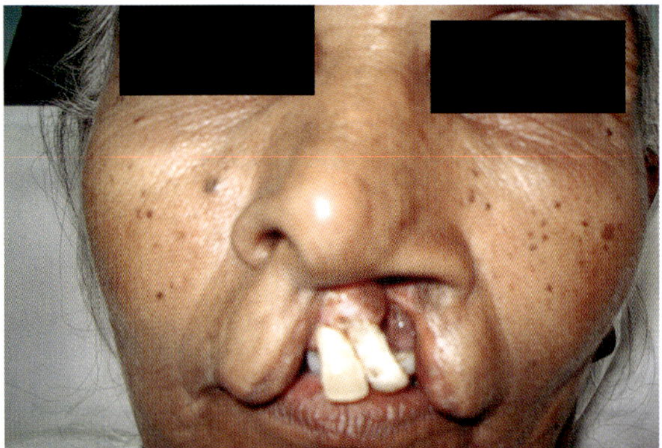

**Fig. 6.16:** A 65-year-old female patient with left unilateral cleft lip

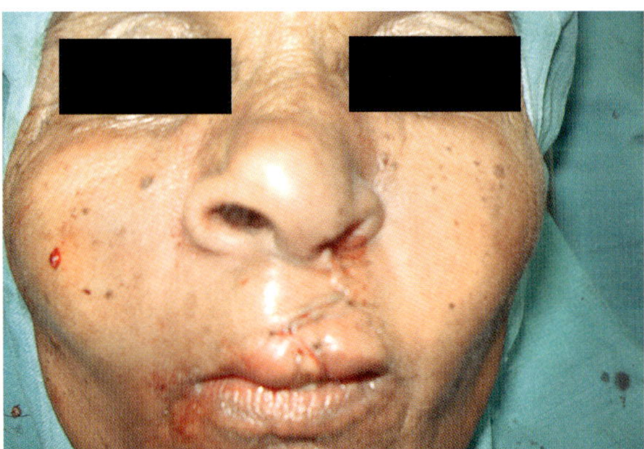

**Fig. 6.17:** Postoperative result of left unilateral cleft lip repair

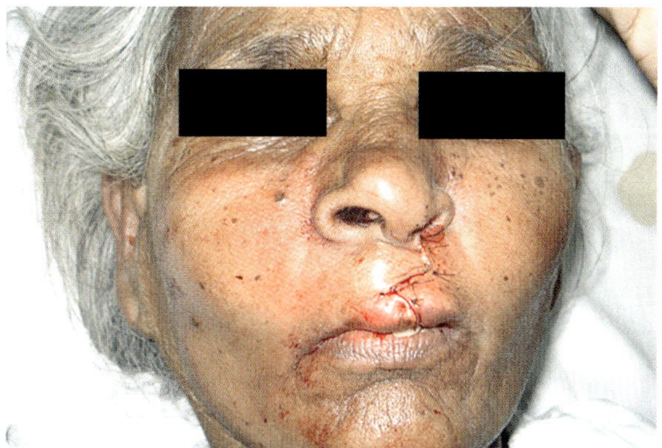

**Fig. 6.18:** Postoperative result of left unilateral cleft lip repair

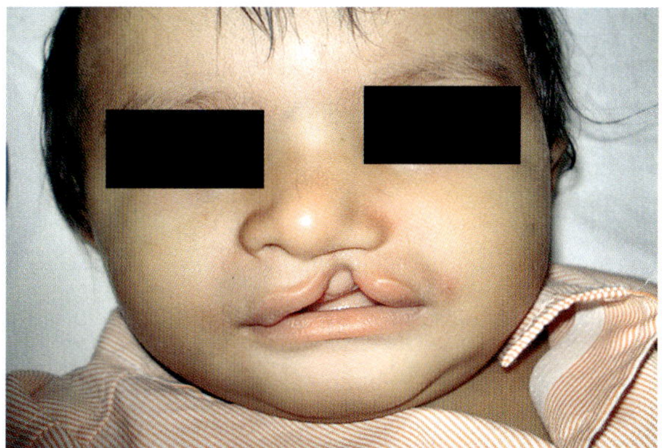

**Fig. 6.19:** Left incomplete unilateral cleft lip

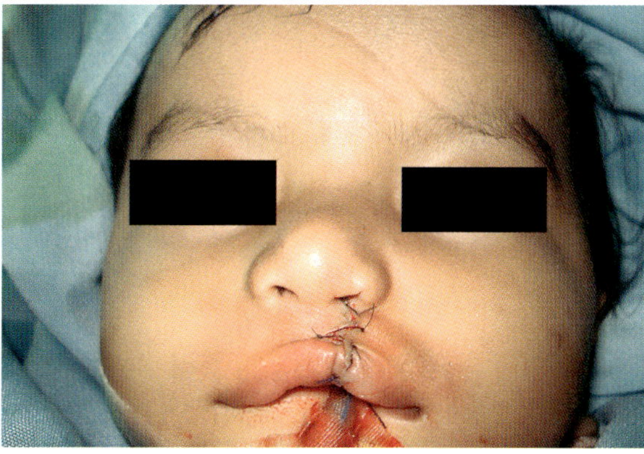

**Fig. 6.20:** Postoperative frontal view of left unilateral cleft lip repair

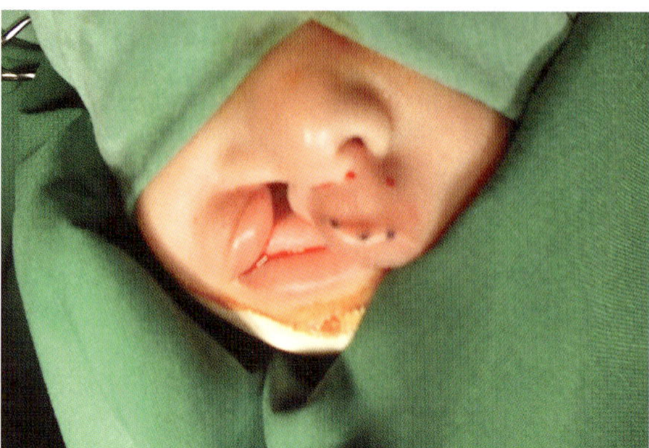

**Fig. 6.21:** Right complete unilateral cleft lip. Three points marked on medial aspect with methylene blue

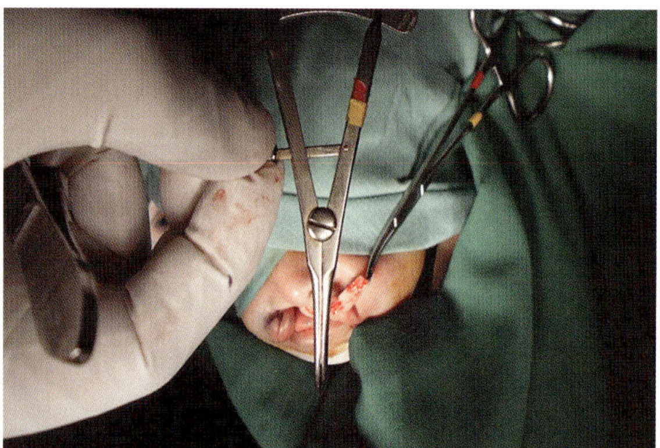

**Fig. 6.22:** Use of calliper for measurement

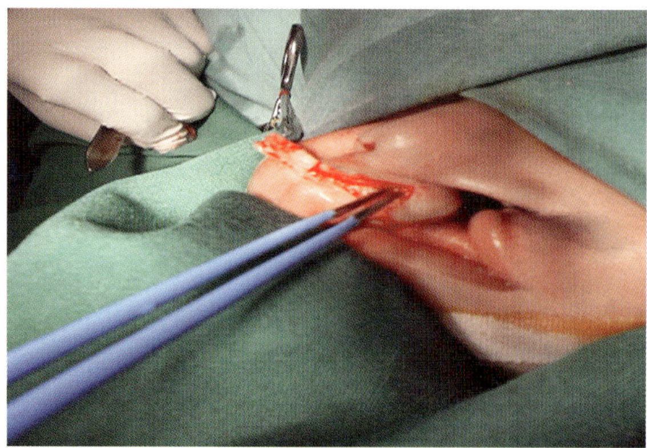

**Fig. 6.23.** Use bipolar cautery for hemostasis

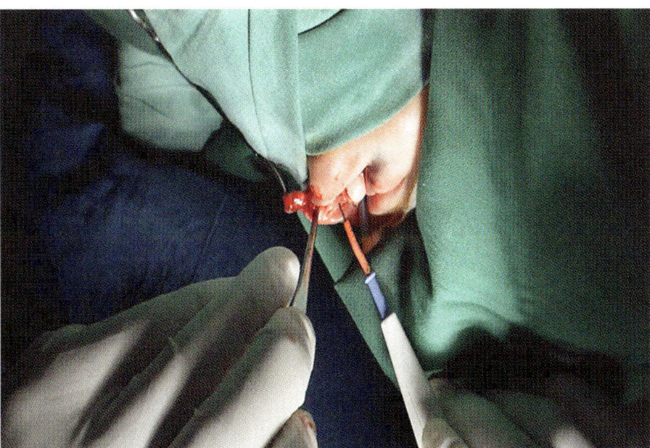

**Fig. 6.24:** Use of monopolar cautery to avoid blood loss particularly over alveolar margin to separate nasal lining

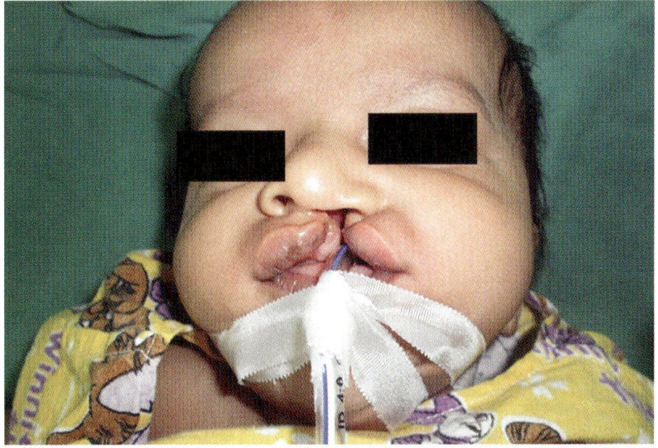

**Fig. 6.25:** Left unilateral cleft lip with palate

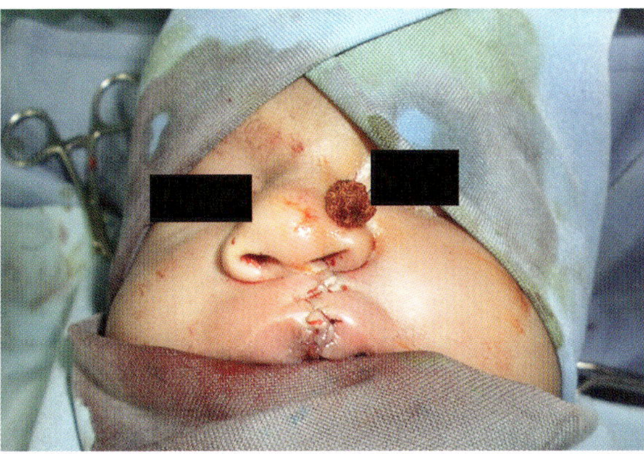

**Fig. 6.26:** Postoperative view of left unilateral cleft lip repair with primary rhinoplasty[27,28]

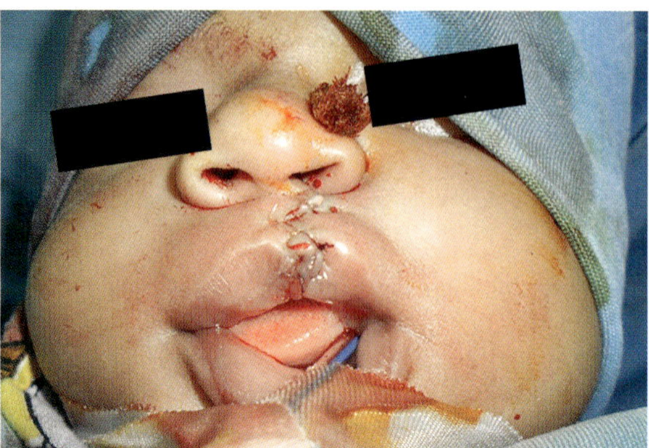

**Fig. 6.27:** Postoperative frontal view

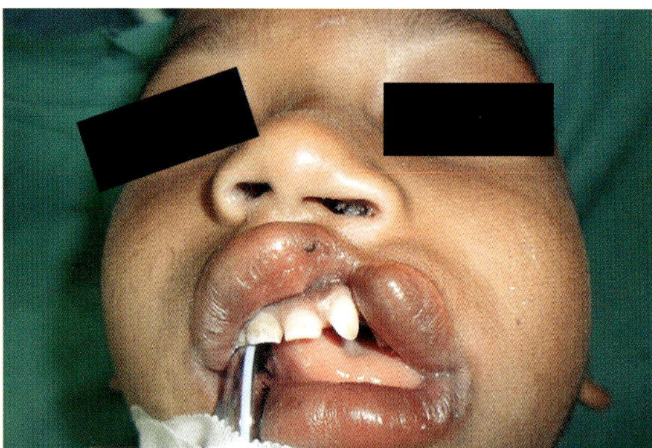

**Fig. 6.28:** Left unilateral cleft lip

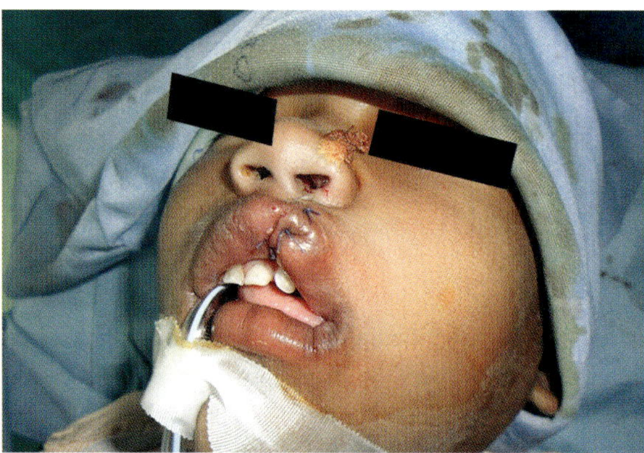

**Fig. 6.29:** Postoperative worms view of left unilateral cleft lip repair

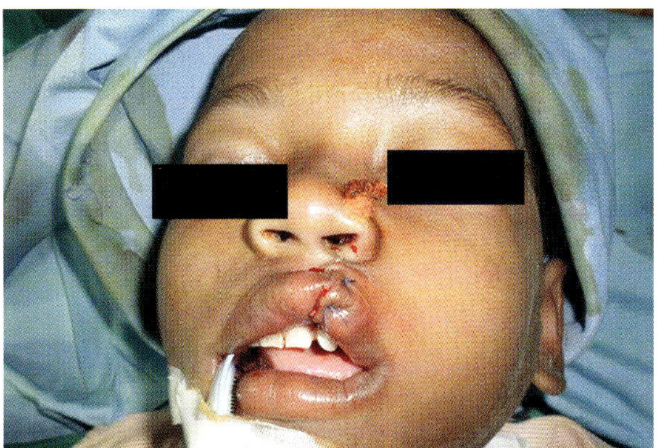

**Fig. 6.30:** Frontal view of left unilateral cleft lip repair

There is no problem in lowering the peak on the medial segment.

This repair has all points according to mathematical pattern. So, it is very easy to learn, perform and teach.

The lengthening of the lip is gained by using a triangular flap[4,29,30] in the lower portion of the lip on the cleft side. This results in minimum tension under the base of the nose.

- So, alar base was placed significantly more lateral and distance from the middome to the lateral alar crease was normal after triangular flap repair in compare to the Millard's rotation and advancement procedure.[31] So later on correction of the nasal deformity was easier.[32]

- $a$, $b$ is a line drawn from the apex of the cupid's bow on the cleft side (equidistance from the midline with that of the noncleft side) to the base of the columella on that side.

- $a$, $b$ less $a$, $b$ equals $x$, the distance that the apex of the cupid's bow must be dropped on the cleft side and equal to the base of the V-flap.

- Points are marked on either side of the cleft in the floor of the cleft nostril (the medial one on a plane with the base of the columella) so that when approximate, the two nostrils will be similar. The point on the lateral side of the nostril floor is marked is marked $b$.

- Where the vermilion the begins to narrow on the lateral side of the cleft, the distance $x$ is measured at a right angle from the mucocutaneous line and $a$ is marked (provisionally).

From the point $b$ a line of length equal to $a$, $b$ is dropped to meet the lateral extent of distance $x$ at $a$. If length $a$, $b$ fails to extend to $a$ that point raised superiorly. In extreme cases a V-wedge is removed just beneath point $b$ to avoid rotating the V-flap off the lip. On the other hand, if length $a$, $b$ extends beyond $a$, this point can be placed more inferiorly.

- A line is dropped from the midpoint of the base of the columella to the midpoint of the cupid's bow. This line is then crossed by a horizontal line passing through the lateral apex of the cupid's bow at $a$, half way from the midpoint of the cupid's bow to the across point of these two lines a point is marked. This point is connected with the apex of the cupid's bow at $a$ and in turn with the point on the medial floor of the nostril to form line of the incision on the medial side of cleft.

- The inferior lap of the medial incision is labeled $y$ and this length is used to form either side of an isosceles triangle on base $x$.
- Measurement of skin envelop of nose was carried out.
- Total nasal length.
- Intercanthal distance.
- Alar to medial canthus on both sides.
- Columellar length both sides.
- Height of dome both sides.
- Distance from intercanthal line to apex on both sides.
- Distance from middome to alar groove on both sides.
- Distance from midcolumella to alar groove on both sides.
- Incisions are carried through the full thickness of the lip along these line located medially and laterally and the lateral V-shaped tonque is introduce into the medial groove, after undermining of the soft tissues and appropriate attension to the nasal deformity.
- Muscles are sutured with 4-0 vicryl.
- Skin edges are sutured with 6-0 ethilon or 5-0 monocryl. Vermilion is sutured 4-0 vicryl.

In the more severe defects a much longer isosceles or even a right triangle of tissue from the upper lateral lip may be utilized. This larger flap provides more tissue and may be carried beyond the midline to lower the midpoint of the cupid's bow if necessary. In such cases the medial incision.

Commencing at point '$A$' will approach the horizontal depending upon the configuration of the V-flap.

## Rotation Advancement Unilateral Cleft Lip Repair[27,28,33-42]

- **Medial incision:** A rotation incision line runs from cleft side cupid bow CPHL upward into the base of columella then turning back to the nasolabial junction of the noncleft side. The C-flap incision runs from CPHL to the lateral point of the skin overlying the premaxilla. C-flap is raised and tip of the C-flap is rotated medially to the columellar base.
- **Lateral incision:** An L-flap extend from maxilla to free border of the lip. Inferior turbinate flap is raised along skin mucosal junction on the pyriform aperture up to the inferior turbinate. A triangular white skin roll flap above CPLH is made.

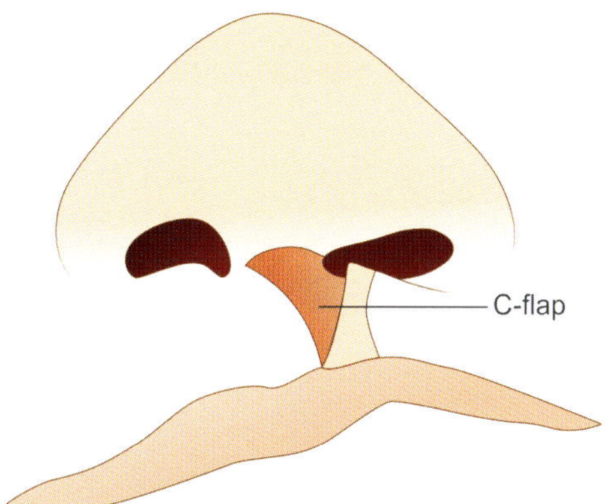


**Fig. 6.31:** Rotation and advancement repair

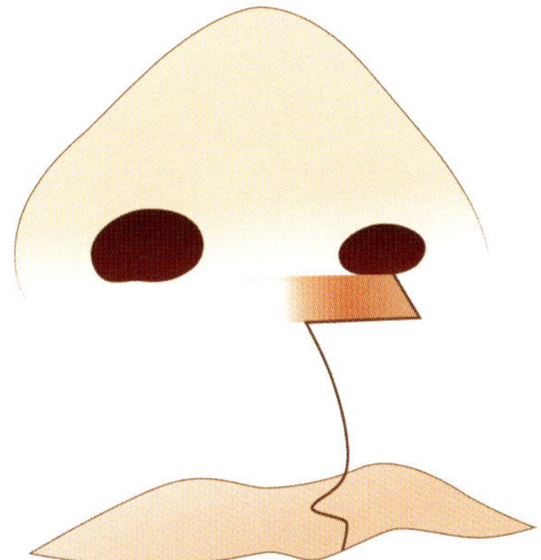

**Fig. 6.32:** Rotation and advancement repair completed

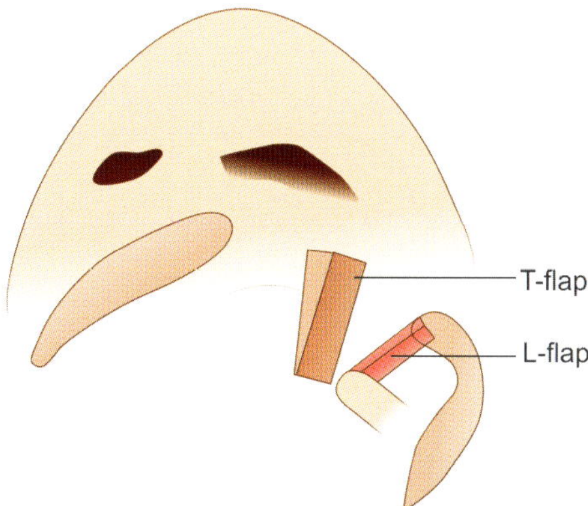


**Fig. 6.33:** The buccal mucosal flap and inferior turbinate flap are elevated based on vestibular lining

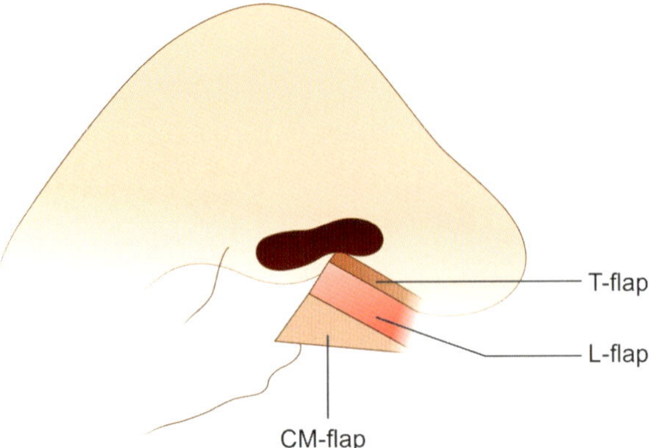


**Fig. 6.34:** Nasal floor reconstruction

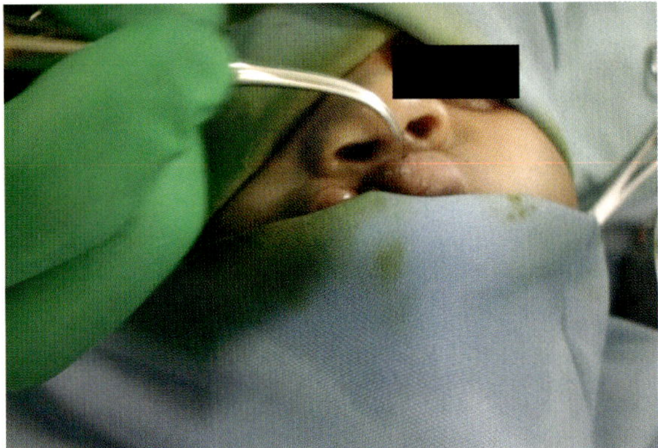

**Fig. 6.35:** Marking of incision is done with methylene blue with use of calliper

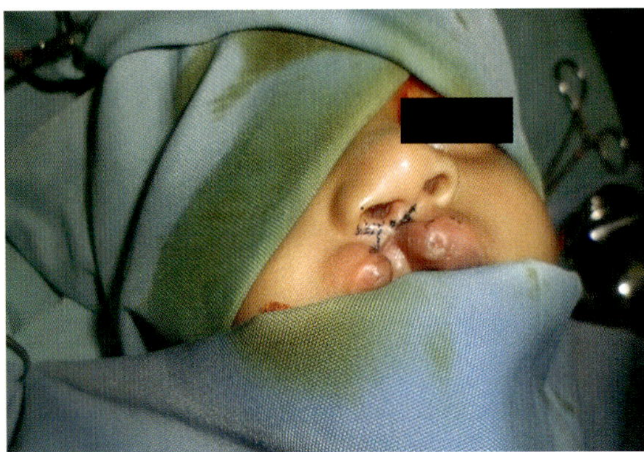

**Fig. 6.36:** Markings done

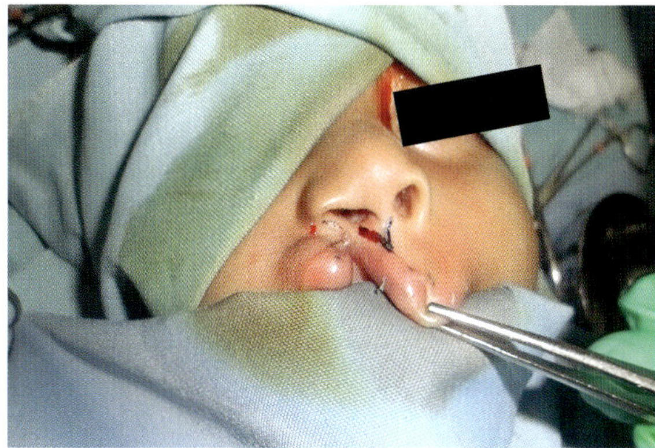

**Fig. 6.37:** Markings on medial and lateral aspect of right unilateral cleft lip

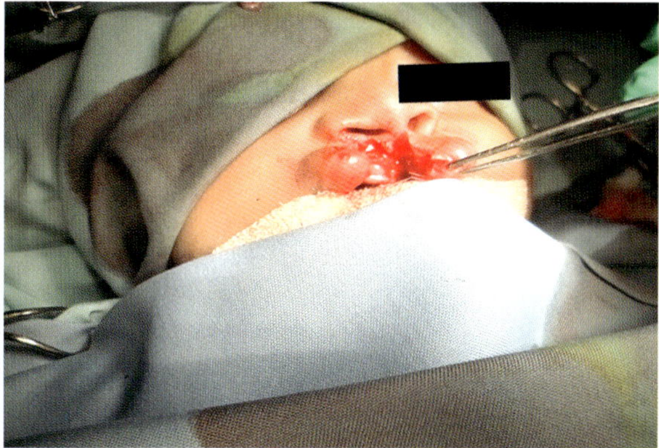

**Fig. 6.38:** Incision kept and dissection done

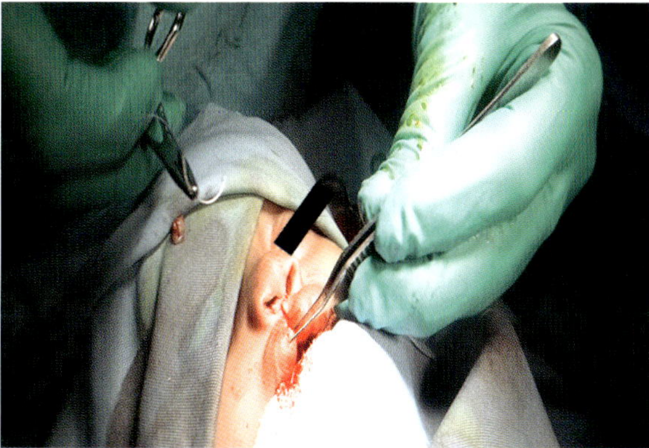

**Fig. 6.39:** Vicryl 4-0 is used for muscle and mucosal repair

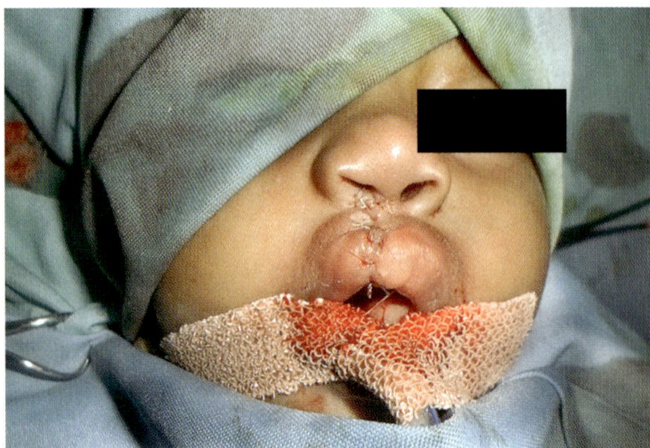

**Fig. 6.40:** Skin was closed with 5-0 monocryl

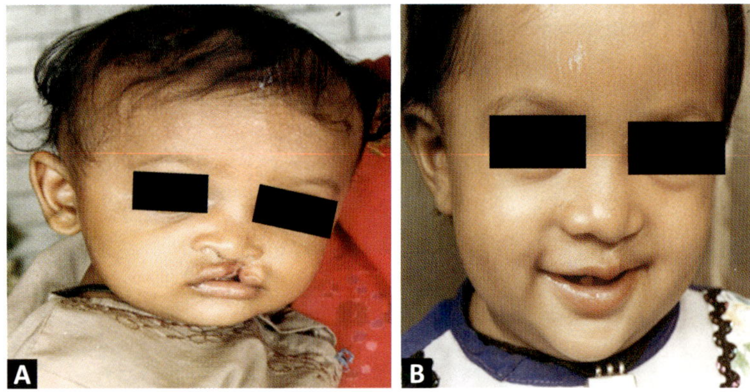

**Figs 6.41A and B:** (A) Left incomplete cleft lip; (B) Postoperative 2 years

- **Nasal floor reconstruction:** The L-flap is sutured to perichondrium behind columella rotating medially. T-flap is sutured to L-flap and C-flap is sutured to L-flap rotating laterally.
- Triangular vermilion flap is marked and incised.
- Muscles are separated from skin for 1–2 mm and sutured with 4-0 vicryl.[13,43] Skin is sutured with 6-0 ethilon or 5-0 monocryl. The small white skin roll flap is sutured to medial lip to reconstruct bulging of white skin roll.
- **Semi-open rhinoplasty:** Rim incision on noncleft side and reversed U-incision is taken on cleft side. The fibrofatty tissue is released from both lower lateral cartilages in nasal tip. Both medial crura of lower.

Lateral cartilages we sutured together with 5-0 prolene. Through and through suture are placed for further support to the lower lateral cartilages. Excessive skin is excised on cleft side to avoid webbing of the soft triangle. Alar base is repositioned by releasing and approximations paranasal muscles. Proper alar facial groove is created by two alar transfixion sutures (Figs 6.31 to 6.40).

## POSTOPERATIVE CARE

To avoid falling back of tongue all the patients were placed in semiprone position immediately after operation, but when this danger is passed away, they were allowed to sleep in supine position.

Boiled water and glucose water orally was started within two hours of the operation and in evening they are were allowed to take normal feed with milk, fruits juices, etc.

To diminish strain on the sutured parts, crying was avoided for several days by possible means.

Splint were given on both upper limbs to all children to avoid interference with suture line.

No sedative were given because in complete cleft lip with cleft of palate, tongue might fall back and cause respiratory obstruction.
Antibiotics were given for five days postoperatively.

### Dressing

After operation nasal cavity on cleft side is packed with vaseline gauze and dry gauze were put over sutureline and micropore applied after retracting cheek towards sutureline. Dressing was done daily. Alternate sutures were removed on the 5th day and remaining on the 7th day with fine instruments.

### Follow Up

The cases were advised follow up after 3 months, 6 months and one year after operation. Thereafter they were followed up once a year (Fig. 6.41).

Cleft palate repair was carried out at age of 9 months. Alar cartilage lift was advised at age of 5 years. Corrective rhinoplasty for deviated nasal septum and nasal bone deformities was deffered till age of 16 years.

For the evaluation of results of surgery, we have examined following features.

- Scar: barely visible
    - Visible
    - Soft and supple
    - Hypertrophy/keloid
    - Widening of scar
    - Line of scar
- Length of the lip, and general contour of the lip
- Cupid's: level
    - Symmetry

- Fullness
- Noticeability

Following features were examined for evaluation of result.

- Sear
- Length of the lip and general contour of the lip
- Cupid's bow
- Vermilion
- Philtrum
- Free border of lip
- Buccal sulcus
- Nostril floor
- Alveolar border.

## REFERENCES


1. Cosman B, Crikelair GF. The shape of the unilateral cleft lip defect. Plastic and Reconstructive Surgery. 1965;35:484-93.
2. Bartels JR, O'Malley JE, Douglas WM, Wilson RG. Variations of masters interlocking Z-cheilorrhaphy. Plast Reconstr Surg. 1970;45(2):189-90.
3. Cardosa AD. A new technique of hare lip. Plast Reconstr Surg. 1952;10:92-5.
4. Cutting CB, Bardach J, Pang R. A comparative study of the skin envelope of the unilateral cleft lip nose subsequent to rotation–advancement and triangular flap lip repairs. Plast Reconstr Surg. 1989;84(3):409-17.
5. Davies D. Transaction of the 5th International Congress of Plastic and Reconstructive Surgery. Melbourne Australia, Buttersworth's. 1971;169-73.
6. Davies D. The repair of unilateral left lip. Br Jr Plast Surg. 1965;18:254-64.
7. DeHaan CR. Initial repair of cleft lip. In: Stark RB, editor. Cleft palate: a multidisciplinary approach. New York: Harper and Row. 1968;113-35.
8. Freedlander E, Webster MH, Lewis RB, Blair M. Knight SL, Brown Al. Neonatal cleft lip repair in Ayshire: a contribution to the debate. Br Jr Plast Surg. 1990;43:197-202.
9. Grabb WC, Smith JW. Plastic surgery 3rd edition, Boston, Little Brown and Co. 1979;193.
10. Grignon JL. Disincertion and rolling up of the ala and lip transposition: Double lock technique for the closure of cleft lip. In: Johanson B. (Ed.) 2nd International Congress on Cleft Palate. Abstracts, Copenhagen. 1973:238.
11. Heckler FR, Oesterle LG, Jabaley ME. The minimal cleft lip revisited-clinical and anatomical correction. Cleft Palate Journal. 1979;16:240.
12. Joos U. Muscle reconstruction in primary cleft lip surgery. J Craniomaxillofac Surg. 1985;15:90-8.
13. Kernahen DA, Bauer BS. Functional cleft lip repair: A sequential, layered closure with orbicularis muscle realignment. Plast Reconstr Surg. 1983;72:459-67.
14. Kernahen DA. Muscle repair in unilateral cleft lip based on findings of electric stimulation. Annals of Plastic Surgery. 978;1:48.
15. Marcks KM. Further observation in cleft lip repair. Plast Reconstr Surg. 1953;12:392.

16. Masters F, Geprgoade N, Horton C, Pickrell K. Use of interlocking Z's in repair of incomplete clefts of lip. Plast Reconstr Surg. 1954;14:287.

17. McCarthy JG. Plastic surgery Philadelphia, WB Saunders and Co. 1990;4.

18. May H. The Axhausen operation for cleft lip repair modified after Hagedorn-LeMesurier principle. Plast Reconstr Surg. 1955;15:21.

19. Randall P. A lip adhesion operation in cleft lip surgery. Plast Reconstr Surg. 1965;35:371.

20. Sawhney CP. Geometry of single cleft lip repair. Plast Surg. 1972;49:518-21.

21. Sharma LK. Primary repair of unilateral cleft lip by triple wedge technique. Indian Journal of Plastic Surgery. 1969;2:39-43.

22. Sinha RN, Gupta JL, Ganguli AC. A textbook of plastic surgery in the tropics. New Delhi: Orient Longman, 14. 1976.

23. Steffenson WH. A method for repair of the unilateral cleft lip. Plast Reconstr Surg. 1949;4:144-52.

24. Skoog T. Repair of unilateral cleft lip deformity maxilla, nose and lip. Scand J Plast Reconstr Surg. 1969;3:109-33.

25. Wynn SK. Lateral flap lip surgery technique. Plast Reconstr Surg. 1960;26:509.

26. Robert F. Hegarty MD. Hegarty's unilateral cleft lip repair surgery. Gyenecology and Obstetrics. 1958:114.

27. Mulliken JB, Martinez-Perez D. The principle of rotation advancement for repair of unilateral complete cleft lip and nasal deformity: technical variations and analysis of results. Plast Reconstr Surg. 1999;104:1247-60.

28. McComb H. Primary correction of unilateral cleft lip nasal deformity: 9-10 years review. Plast Reconstr Surg. 1985;75:791-9.

29. Cronin TD. A modification of Tennison-type lip repair. Cleft Palate J. 1966;3:376-82.

30. Saunders DE, Malek A, Karandy E. Growth of the cleft lip following a triangular flap repair. Plast Reconstr Surg. 1986;72(2):227-38.

31. Barbel MD, Holtmann, Wray, R Chris MD. A Randomized comparison of triangular and rotation—advancement unilateral cleft lip repairs. Plastic and Reconstructive Surgery. 1983;71:171-8.

32. Callister AC. Technique designed to prevent lateral creeping of alar cartilage in repair of hare-lip. Plast Reconstr Surg. 1948;3(5):617-20.

33. Millard DR. Cleft craft. Boston: Little Brown and Co. 1976;1.

34. Millard DR, Latham R, Huifen X, et al. Cleft lip and palate treated by presurgical orthopaedics, gingivoperiosteoplasty, and lip adhesion compared with previous lip adhesion method; preliminary study of serial dental casts. Plast Reconstr Surg. 1999;103:1630-44.

35. Nicolau PJ. The orbicularis oris muscle: A functional approach to its repair in cleft lip. Br Jr plast Surg. 1983;36:141.

36. Noordhof MS, Chen PKT. Unilateral cheiloplasty. In: Mathes ST (ed.) Plastic Surgery. Philadelphia: WB Saunders; 2006;4.

37. Noordoff MS, Chen YR, Chen KT, et al. The surgical technique for the complete unilateral cleft lip—nasal deformity. Plast Reconstr Surg. 1995;2:167-74.

38. Peet EW. Cleft lip and palate. In: Rob C, Smith R. Eds. Operative Surgery, Philadelphia: Lippincot. 1969;75-97.

39. Pool R. The configurations of the unilateral cleft lip, with reference to the rotation advancement repair. Plast Reconstr Surg. 1966;37:558-65.

40. Salyer KE. Early and late treatment of unilateral cleft nasal deformity. Cleft Palate Craniofac J. 1992;29:556-69.
41. Thomson HJ. Clinical evaluation of microform cleft lip surgery. Plast Reconstr Surg. 1985;75:800-3.
42. Williams HB. A Method of assessing cleft lip repair: Comparison of LeMesurier and Millard technique. Plast Reconstr Surg. 1968;41:1103.
43. Bardach J. Discussion: the effect of cleft lip repair on maxillary morphology in patients with unilateral complete cleft lip and palate. Plast Reconstr Surg. 1996;97: 1376-8.

# CHAPTER 7

# Bilateral Cleft Lip Repair

## INTRODUCTION

The different embryological theories like failure in the fusion of Dursy and His or failure of the mesodermal migration of Fleischmann-Veau-Stark or failure of the merging of Patten or combination of these, whatever fail on one side in unilateral cleft lip fail on both sides in bilateral cleft lip/palate. The primary palate and the secondary palate are delineated by the incisive foramen as the central landmark and suture extending anterolaterally to the spaces between the maxillary lateral incisor and the first canine tooth on both side. Primary palate comprises central portion of the upper lip, premaxilla, upper incisors and anterior nasal septum, forms between the fourth and seventh weeks of intrauterine life and extend to the nasopalatine canal site of the incisive foramen. The secondary palate comprising the remainder the hard palate and the soft palate posterior to the incisive foramen forms between seventh and twelfth weeks as a pair of shelves that grows towards midline and fuse in normal embryo. There is no muscle fibers in the prolabium of complete bilateral clefts. Premaxilla develops from two pairs of the ossification centers. The principal pair forms primordia of the lateral incisors, extend upward and with the maxilla proceeds forward to embrace the premaxilla on either side. The union is complete by the end of the third month. Protrusion of premaxilla in bilateral cleft lip begins at about 45 days and then develops rapidly for 25 days to reach proportion at 70 days comparable to those seen at birth. The anatomical incompleteness and functional inefficiency of the musculus oris in complete bilateral clefts contributes the most probably to the formation of the protrusion of the premaxilla. The premaxillary segment is under no restrain laterally either forms bone or gingival fibrous tissue, consequently its attachment to the nasal saptum by septomaxillary legament becomes dominant factor. As the nasal septum grows forward it draws the upper jaw with it but not at the same rate. In the bilateral cleft premaxillary segment is carried forward at the same rate as that of the growing septum to which it is firmly held.

In unilateral cleft, the premaxilla is normally attached to the maxilla on one side and this entire component is rotated outward varying degrees from the cleft side maxilla in an asymmetrical distortion. Bilateral clefts present an entirely different configuration. In the complete bilateral cleft, the premaxilla is unattached to either maxilla, thus there are three separate components which are more or less symmetrical in their distortion. The two maxillae are usually equal to each other in size and position while the central premaxilla element proceed forwards on its own, in different degrees but with symmetry within itself except for possible deviation. The complete separation of the central frontonasal component of prolabium and premaxilla from lateral maxillary segments abnormally influences the nose, philtrum, musculation, vascularity, nerve supply, growth and development of three elements. Where the cleft is incomplete on both sides the deformity is less and still symmetrical. In such a case, there is usually a more or less intact alveolus and little or no protrusion of the premaxilla.[1,2] The columella is likely to be longer than in the complete cleft but not of normal length.[3,4] Sometimes, the degree of the cleft varies on each side. Sometimes the degree of the incompleteness shows as only the slightest notch on one side and halfway or three quarter cleft on opposite side. There can be a complete cleft on one side and an incomplete on the other side. Residual congenital skin bridges spanning the upper portion of lip clefts are known as Simonart's bands. Yuzuriha and Mulliken classified bilateral incomplete cleft lips in minor forms, microform and minimicroform. The skin of the prolabium is thin with scanty or no hairs. The median tubercle constains the right and left premaxilla united by a median sutures. Each premaxilla is enlarged laterally to carry two incisor teeth, a central incisor looking inferolaterally and lateral incisor at a higher level looking posterolaterally. Extending posteriorly as an extension from the premaxilla is the subvomerine process which produces a groove. In this rests the cartilaginous nasal septum and the long and narrow vomer. The prolabium is the soft tissue end point of the frontonasal component. Prolabium may vary in size from a few millimeters to over a centimeter in height and width.

In bilateral cleft lip, it is shortened possessing neither Cupid's bow, nor philtrum columns, nor labial sulcus and is attached to little or no columella. In the complete bilateral cleft, the superior labial artery fails to unite with its fellow from the opposite side and does not contribute to philtrum. In addition to this, the arcade made up by the anastomosis of the posterior septal branch with the greater palatine artery through the incisive foramen is absent.

The philtrum and premaxilla derive their blood supply from posterior septal artery, lateral nasal artery and terminal branch of anterior ethmoidal vessels which pass through the columella.

Pierre Franco described primary excision of the projecting premaxilla and sutured prolabium laterally. Guillaume Dupuytren excised premaxilla and used prolabium for columellar reconstruction. Johan Philip Hoffman described compressive bandages for pressure over projecting premaxilla in 1686, and later on compressive garment were modified by Louis, Desault,

Malgango and Hulliben in late 18th century. Mladick and Thorne suggested K-wire for controlled fixed external traction, Latham and Georgiade promoted pinned coaxial screw appliances in 1975. Gensoul sized the projecting premaxilla with a strong forceps and forced it back with sufficient strength to fracture the vomer.[5] Adolf von Bardeleben as first to section the vomer subperiosteally in 1865. Veau, Browne, Cronin[6] and Monroe described their own methods for resection of vomer for premaxilla setback. Technique desribed for unilateral cleft lip repair were modified for bilateral cleft lip repair.[7,8] Lip was repair initially on one side after 3–6 months, but this led to asymmetry of look on both sides. Rectangular flaps from lateral elements were inserted beneath the prolabium by Konig, Hagedorn, Mirault and Barsky. Triangular flap or quadrilateral flaps from lateral labial elements were interdigited into prolabium.[9] These methods resulted into long lip vertically and tight lip horizontally. Philtrum has a remarkable capacity for vertical growth once it is attached to the lateral labial elements.

Veau III[7,10,11] straight line repair and its modification became the standard design, but these methods lacked muscle repair. Manchester[8] attached muscles to the side of prolabium to avoid pressure over premaxilla. Millard repair involved complete elevation of prolabium and repaired muscle.[12,13] Millard banked lateral segments of prolabium as forked flap for columellar reconstruction later on. Schultz, Browne, Glover and McComb advocated primary muscle repair to minimize lateral drift of the alar base and widening of the philtrum. McComb[14-17] described primary rhinoplasty with bilateral cleft lip repair.[18-20]

## OPERATION (FIGS 7.1 TO 7.18)

Under general anesthesia with noncuffed oral RAE endotracheal tube and throat pack, patient is kept supine with neck extended position. Marking is done with methylene blue dye. Local xylocaine with adrenaline is injected. Prolabial flap is made. Flap is tie-shaped, broad bellow and narrow above near columella. De-epithelization is done on lateral segment of prolabium. In cases were prolabium is very narrow we recommend de-epithelization of lateral labial segment for better cosmetic outcome. Lateral lip incision is kept. The peak of the Cupid's bow is determined where the dry vermilion is maximal in width before it tapers off superiorly. Incision extends from vermilion cutaneous junction to the alar base. The incision extends to intranasally along the mucocutaneous junction. The vermilion of the lateral flap will fit into the inferior edge of the prolabial flap and to each other in midline forming a tubercle. The white roll should be included in the vermilion flaps. Muscle is separated from skin and mucosa for 1–2 mm. Upper buccal incision is made for mobilization. Alar bases are freed from their attachments to the piriform region for medial and inferior mobilization. The lower lateral cartilages are freed from overlying nasal skin through infracartilaginous incision medially and laterally. Intradomal sutures are taken for approximation of the dome and complex is suspended to upper lateral cartilage with temporary fixation sutures. Labial sulcus is created by approximating the labial mucosa of the lateral lip elements to the turned over central labial mucosa. Orbicularis oris muscles[21,22] are sutured with 4-0 vicryl and skin sutured 6-0 ethilon sutures (Figs 7.19 to 7.21).

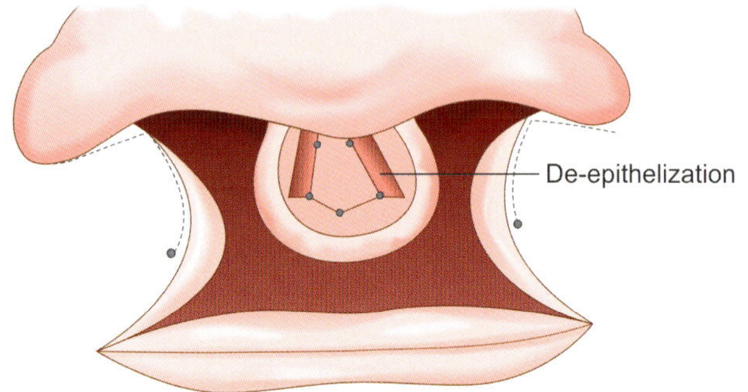


**Fig. 7.1:** Mulliken's repair[10,11,23-27]

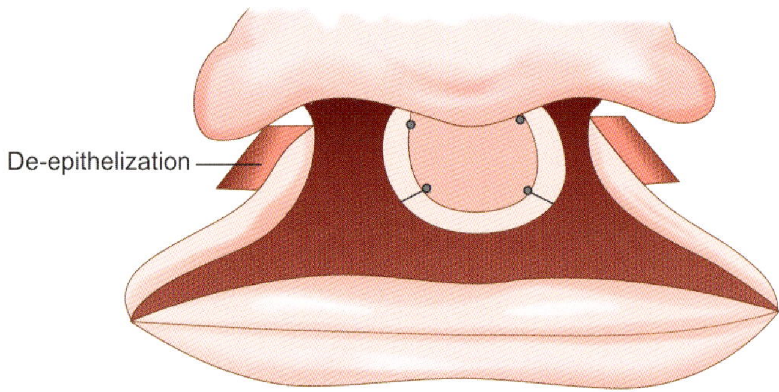


**Fig. 7.2:** Veau-III repair[28]

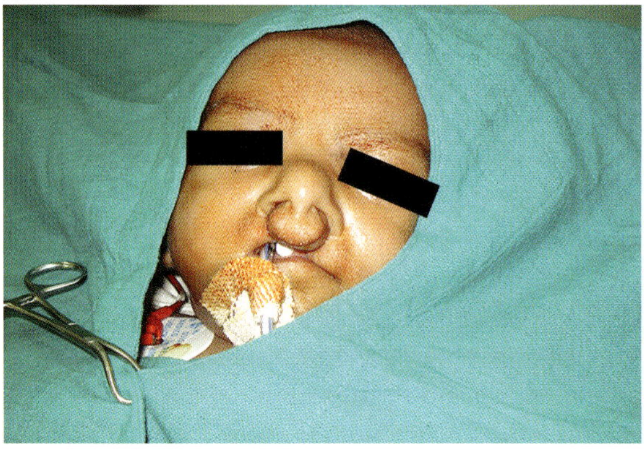

**Fig. 7.3:** Patient with bilateral cleft lip with palate

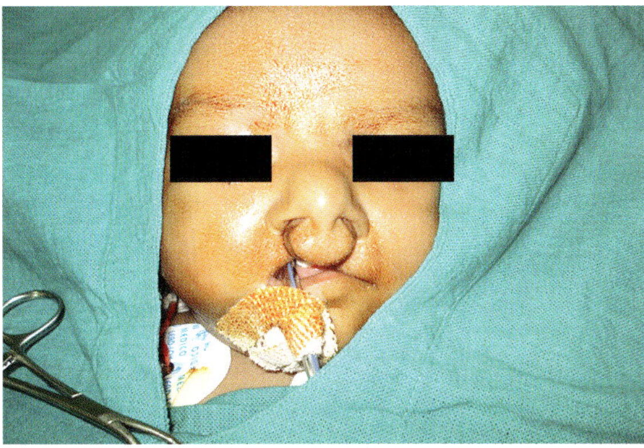

**Fig. 7.4:** Front view of patient with bilateral cleft lip and palate

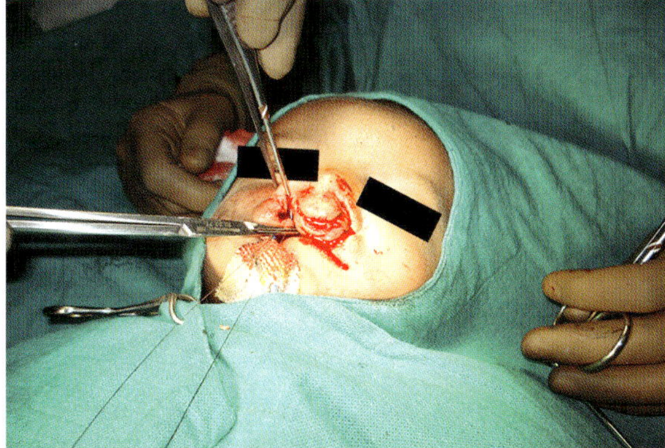

**Fig. 7.5:** Veau-III repair incision was placed. De-epithelization was done in lateral segments

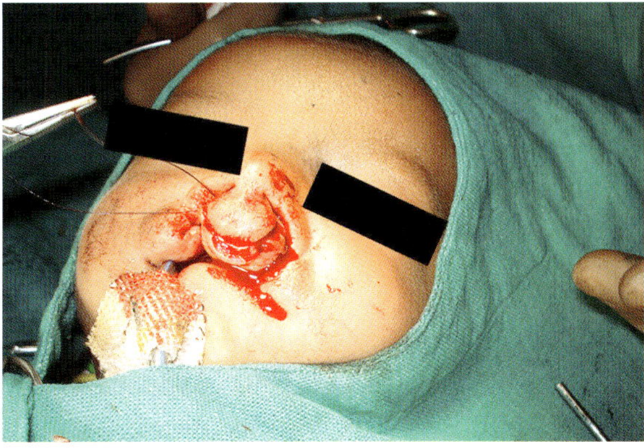

**Fig. 7.6:** Muscle are repaired with 4-0 vicryl

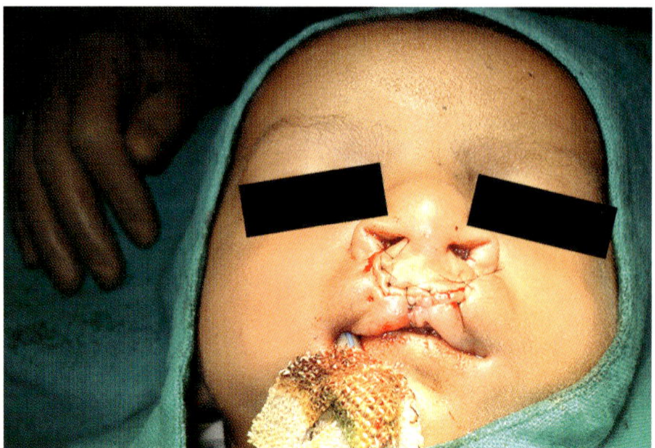

**Fig. 7.7:** Skin closure was done with 6-0 nylon suture

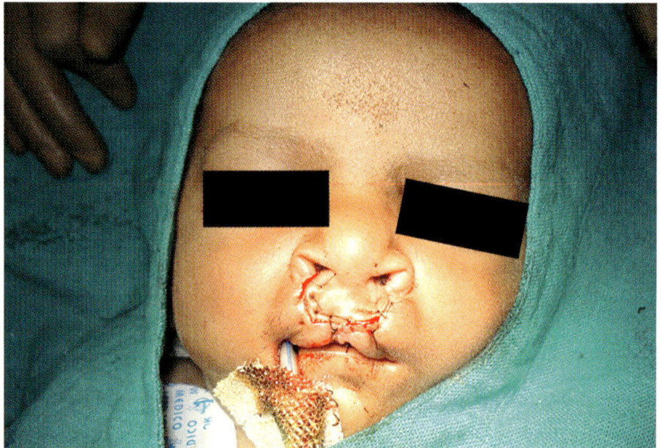

**Fig. 7.8:** Front view of completed repair of bilateral cleft lip

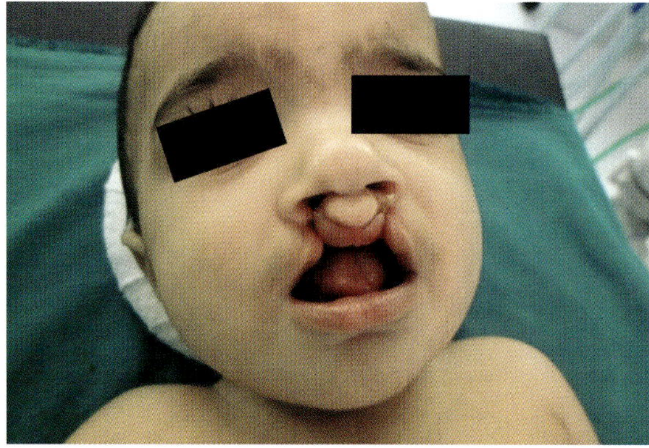

**Fig. 7.9:** Patient is having bilateral cleft lip with cleft palate

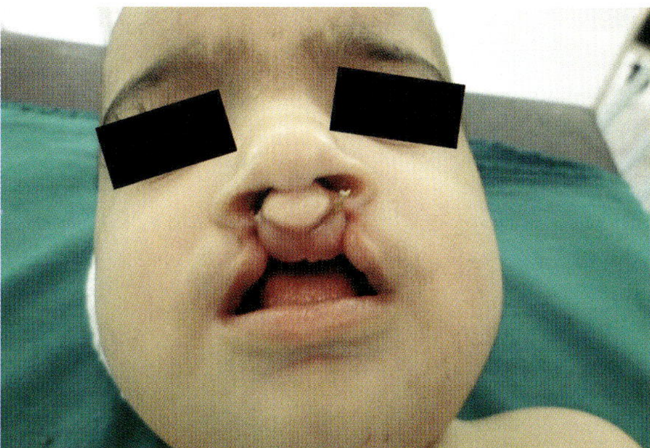

**Fig. 7.10:** Worms view of patient with bilateral cleft lip and palate

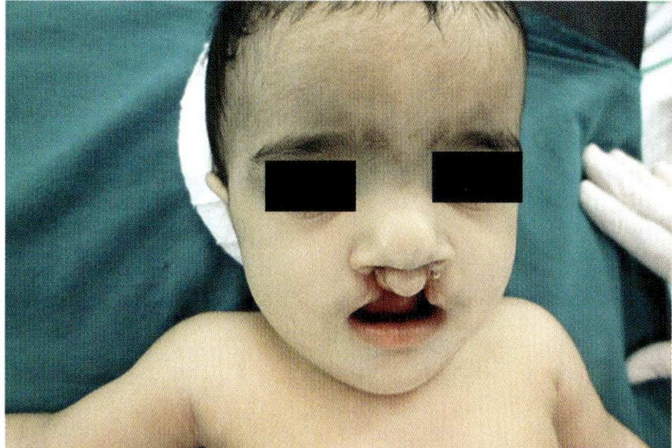

**Fig. 7.11:** Bilateral cleft lip with palate

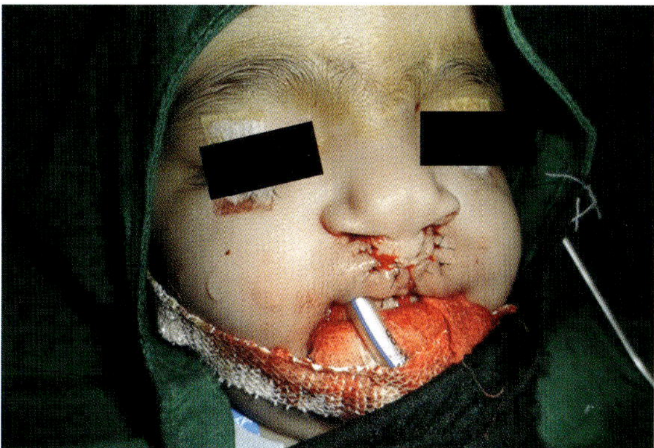

**Fig. 7.12:** Mucosa and muscles were repaired with 4-0 vicryl and skin closed with 6-0 nylon

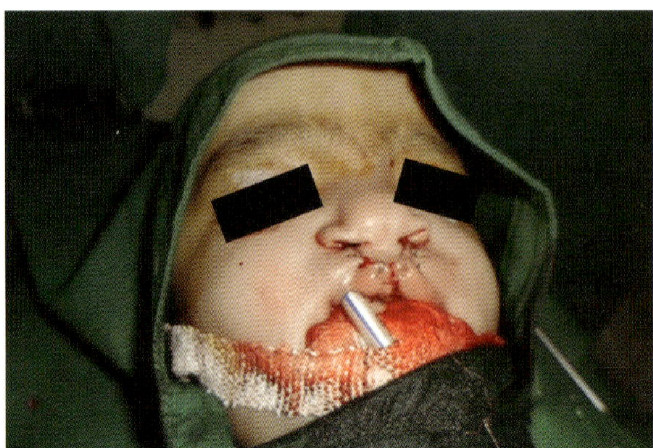

**Fig. 7.13:** Worms view of completed bilateral cleft lip repair

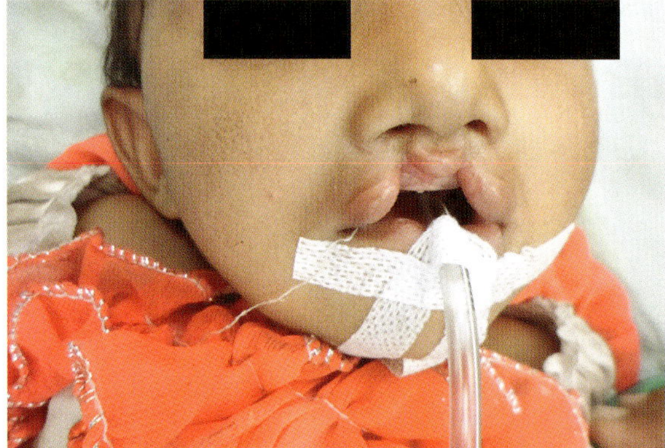

**Fig. 7.14:** Patient with bilateral cleft lip with palate. Prolabium is narrow and short

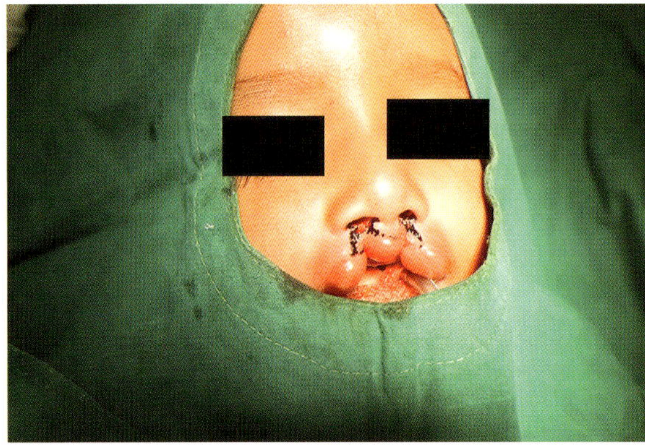

**Fig. 7.15:** Veau-III repair is planned

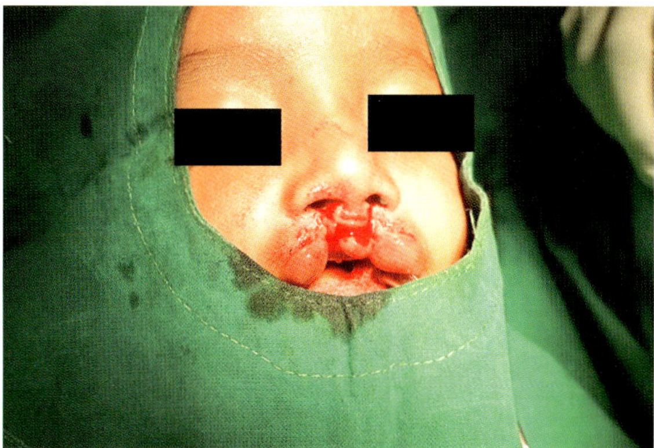

**Fig. 7.16:** Incision were kept, de-epithelization was done on lateral segments

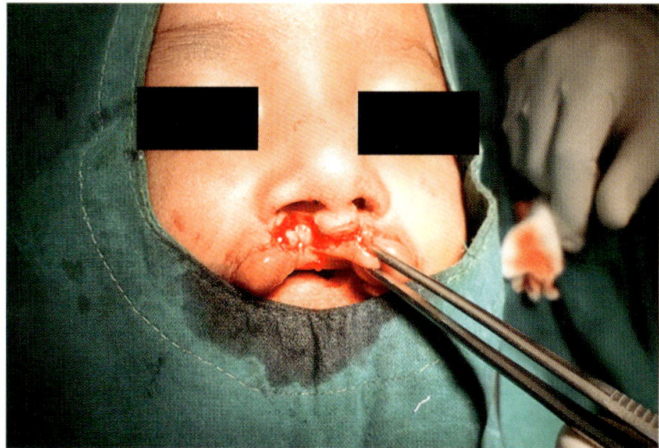

**Fig. 7.17:** Muscle and mucosa were sutured with 4-0 vicryl

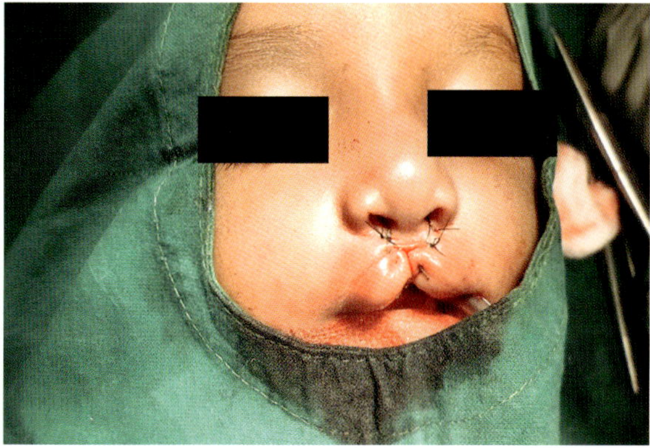

**Fig. 7.18:** Skin was sutured with 6 0 nylon

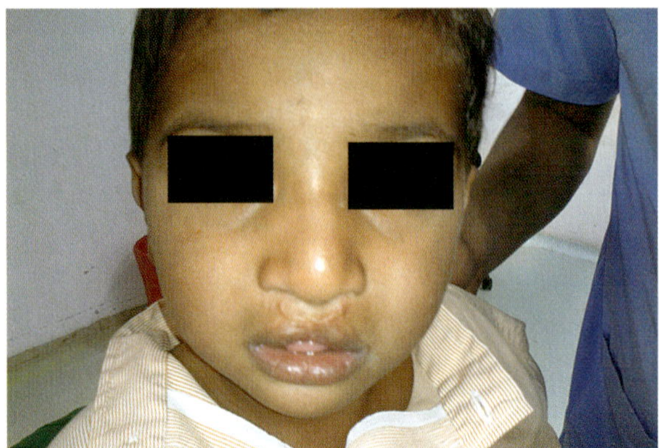

**Fig. 7.19:** Patient with repaired bilateral cleft lip with Veau-III repair after two years of surgery[7]

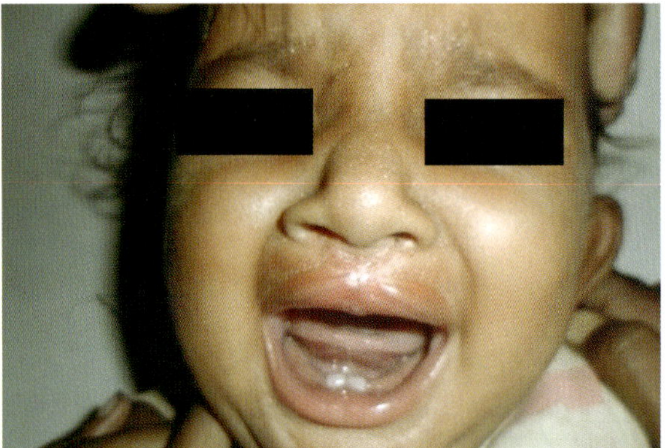

**Fig. 7.20:** Patient with repaired bilateral cleft lip with Mulliken repair after 6 months of surgery

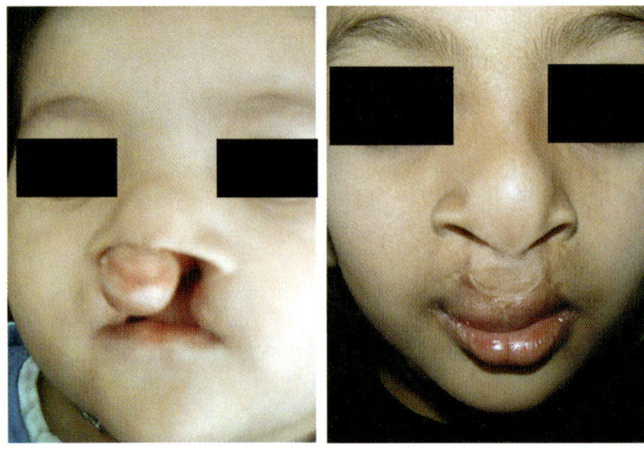

**Fig. 7.21:** Bilateral cleft lip repair follow up after 6 years

## REFERENCES


1. Broadbent TR, Woolf RM. Cleft lip nasal deformity. Ann Plast Surg. 1984;12(3):216-34.
2. Lee CT, Garfinkle JS, Warren SM, et al. Nasoalveolar molding improves appearance of children with bilateral cleft lip-cleft palate. Plast Reconstr Surg. 2008;122:1131-7.
3. Cutting C, Grayson B, Brecht L, et al. Presurgical columellar elongation and primary retrograde nasal reconstruction in one-stage bilateral cleft lip and nose repair. Plast Reconstr Surg. 1998;101:630-9.
4. Yuzuriha S, Oh AK, Mulliken JB. Asymmetrical bilateral cleft lip: complete or incomplete and contralateral lesser defect (minor-form, microform, or mini-microform). Plast Reconstr Surg. 2008;122:1494-504.
5. Monroe CW. Recession of the premaxilla in bilateral cleft lip and palate: A follow up study. Plast Reconstr Surg. 1965;35:512-30.
6. Cronin TD. Lengthening columella by use of skin from nasal floor and alae. Plast Reconstr Surg. 1958;21:417-26.
7. Bitter K. Repair of bilateral cleft lip, alveolus and palate. Part 3: Follow-up criteria and late results. J Maxillofac Surg. 2001;29(1):49-55.
8. Manchester W. The repair of bilateral cleft lip and palate. Br J Surg. 1965;52:878-82.
9. Skoog T. The management of the bilateral cleft of the primary palate (lip and alveolus): General consideration and soft tissue repair. Plast Reconstr Surg. 1965;35:34-44.
10. Mulliken JB. Bilateral cleft lip. Clin Plast Surg. 2004;31:209-20.
11. Mulliken JB. Principles and techniques of bilateral complete cleft lip repair. Plast Reconstr Surg.1985;75:477-86.
12. Millard Jr DR. Columella lengthening by a forked flap. Plast Reconstr Surg. 1958;21:454-7.
13. Millard Jr DR. Cleft craft : The evoluation of its surgery, vol.2 Boston Little, brown 1977.
14. McComb HK. Primary repair of the bilateral cleft lip nose: A long term follow-up. Plast Reconstr Surg. 2009;124:1610-5.
15. McComb H. Primary repair of the bilateral cleft lip nose: A 4 years review. Plast Reconstr Surg. 1994;94:37-47.
16. McComb H. Primary repair of the bilateral cleft lip nose: A 10 years review. Plast Reconstr Surg. 1986;77:701-13.
17. McComb H. Primary repair of the bilateral cleft lip nose. Br J Plast Surg. 1975;28:262-7.
18. Noordhoff MS. Bilateral cleft lip reconstruction. Plast Reconstr Surg. 1986;78:45-54.
19. Stark RB. The development of centre of face with particular reference to surgical correction of bilateral cleft lips. Plast Reconstr Surg. 1958;21:177-92.
20. Troft JA, Mohan N. A preliminary report on one stage open tip rhinoplasty at the time of lip repair in bilateral cleft lip and palate: The Alor Setar experience. Br J. Plast Surg. 1993;46:215-22.
21. Duffy MM. Restoration of orbicularis oris muscle continuity in the repair of the bilateral cleft lip. Br J Plast Reconstr Surg. 1971;24:48-56.

22. Nagase T, Januszkiewicz JS, Keall HJ, et al. The effect of muscle repair on postoperative facial skeletal growth in children with bilateral cleft lip and palate. Scand J Plast Reconstr Surg Hand Surg. 1998;32:395-405.
23. Kim SK, Lee JH, Lee KC, et al. Mulliken method of bilateral cleft lip repair. anthropometric evaluation. Plast Reconstr Surg. 2005;116:1243-51.
24. Morovic CG, Cutting C. Combining the Cutting and Mulliken methods for primary repair of the bilateral cleft lip nose. Plast Reconstr Surg. 2005;116:1613-9.
25. Mulliken JB, Wu JK, Padwa BL. Repair of bilateral cleft lip; review, revision and reflections. J Craniofac Surg. 2003;14:609-20.
26. Mulliken JB. Correction of the bilateral cleft lip nasal deformity : evoluation of a surgical concept. Cleft Palate Craniofac J. 1992;29:540-5.
27. Mulliken JB. Bilateral complete cleft lip and nasal deformity: An anthropometric analysis of staged to synchronous repair. Plast Reconstr Surg. 1995;96:9-23.
28. Veau V. operative treatment of complete double harelip. Ann Surg. 1922;76:143-56.

# CHAPTER 8

# Cleft Palate Repair

Anterior portion of hard palate mucosa has an irregular surface covered by rugae while the posterior portion of the hard palate and soft palate are covered by smooth mucosal surface.

The incisive papillae lies posterior to the alveolar ridge and median raphe extend from incisive papilla to the uvula. Tonsillar pillars lies on posterolateral walls of the oral cavity on each side. The palatoglossal muscle forms anterior pillar and the palatopharyngeal muscle form posterior pillar. A horizontal Passavant ridge may be noted on the posterior wall of pharynx. This ridge is formed by the superior pharyngeal constrictor or horizontal fibers of the palatopharyngeus muscle. The hard palate has keratinized stratified squamous epithelium. The soft palate has nonkeratinized stratified squamous epithelium on the oral surface and pseudostratified ciliated columnar epithelium on nasal surface. The anterior portion of the hard palate is formed by palatine process of the maxilla and posterior portion of hard palate is formed by the horizontal laminae of the palatine bone. The greater palatine and lesser palatine foramine containing the greater and lesser neurovascular bundle are located in the posterolateral portion of bone. Vomer is attached posterior to palatine bone. The sphenoid lies posterior to the palatine bones and has two vertical processes, the medial and lateral pterygoid plates. The pterygoid hamulus extends from the inferior portion of the medial pterygoid plate and serve as a pulley for the tensor veli palatini muscle. The temporal bone is posterolateral to sphenoid bone and contains the orifice to the bony portion of the Eustachian tube. The cartilaginous portion extend from bony portion to inferior, medial and anterior to the pharynx. The opening of Eustachian tube is just above the level of the hard palate on lateral pharyngeal wall. The torus tubarius is an in-bulging of the pharyngeal wall posterior to the tubal opening.

The muscle in the velopharyngeal region[1] plays important role in swallowing, speech production and auditory tube function. The extrinsic muscles of the palate are levetor veli palatini, tensor veli palatini, palatoglossus, palatopharyngeus, salpingopharyngeus, and superior constrictor have a origin or insertion in palate. The only intrinsic muscle is the musculus uvulae. The levetor veli  palatini is a cylindrical muscle. It forms a sling that suspends the soft palate from the cranial base (Figs 8.1 and 8.2). It arises from posteromedial part of  the  Eustachian tube at the junction of its cartilaginous and bony portions. The muscle descends on each side anteriorly and medially toward the soft palate between superior constrictor and the cranial base. The levator enters the velum by fanning out and lies between two heads of the palatopharyngeus. The fibers spread over the posterior three fourth in the velum. Levator occupies middle 50% of the velar length. This fibers  cross midline to meet fibers of opposite levator muscle. Levator muscle are attached anteriorly to the posterior margin of the aponeurosis of the tensor veli palatini. Levator veli palatini is the most superior muscle within soft palate except musculus uvulae. The levator

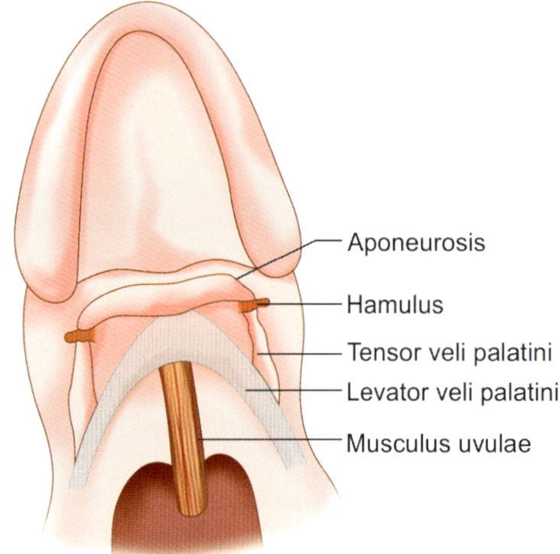


**Fig. 8.1:** Muscles of normal palate

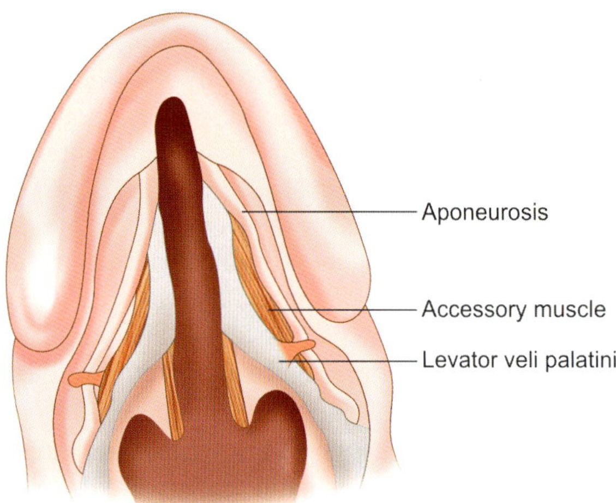


**Fig. 8.2:** Dearranged muscle in cleft palate

veli palatini is thin and hypoplastic in cleft palate. The posterior bundles run posterolaterally towards the palatopharyngeus and medial bundles radiate into the margin of the cleft. The anterior bundles are either attached to the triangular tendinous area of the posterior edge of the palate or directly linked to the tendon of the tensor veli palatini. The function of levator is velar elevation and retrodisplacement during speech and swallowing. Levator veli palatini causes an upward, medial and posterior displacement of the medial tubal cartilage by muscle isotonic contraction with a superior and posterior displacement of the levator sling, resulting in the opening of the lumen of the Eustachian tube.[2,3] It also dilate membranous part of the Eustachian tube. Serous otitis  media in patients with cleft palate is due to dysfunction of the paratubal muscles, particularly the levator veli palatini. The ability of the levator veli palatini to dilate the Eustachian tube is lost in the unrepaired cleft due to its substantial anterior bony insertion on the posterior margin of the hard palate. Repositioning of the levator veli palatini during an intervelar veloplasty and the Furlow double opposing Z-plasty restore the velar suspensory apparatus, allowing dilatation of the Eustachian tube. The tensor veli palatini[4] arises from the scaphoid fossa of the greater wing of the sphenoid between the superior end of the medial pterygoid plate and the spine of the sphenoid as well as the adjacent superolateral aspect of the cartilaginous and membranous part of the entire length of the Eustachian tube. The muscle is triangular with a fleshy belly and tendinous at both ends. It lies at 30–40° with Eustachian tube. The tendon of the tensor  veli palatini hookes around the anterior aspect of the hamulus to enter soft palate at ninety degree. The tendon spread to became the horizontal sheet like aponeurosis occupying the anterior quarter of the velar length. The tensor veli palatini is thinner in cleft patients. Few fibers are attached to the hamulus. The front parts of its bundles extend along the rudimentary palatine aponeurosis towards the posterior nasal spine or run laterally to the posterior edge of the palatine bone. The main tendon archs backward to the cleft margin and ends into two different manners. (1) The tendon occasionally is partially dispersed and a triangular portion passes into the anterior bundles of the levator; (2) The tendon does not disperse and passes anteriorly into the levator veli palatini to form a thick muscular tendinous bundle. The tensor veli palatini dilate Eustachian tube by pulling it inferiorly, laterally and anteriorly. Along with  levator veli palatini tensor augments the opening and may have pumping action that milks the tube of its contents. Complete hamulus fracture reduces the effectiveness of tubal dilatation by the tensor veli palatini. The musculus uvulae is paired muscle running longitudinally in the nasal midline of the velum. It is attached anteriorly to aponeurosis and posteriorly to the base of uvula. The uvula is devoid of muscle fibers. The musculus uvulae is the patella of the levator knee. It increases its diameters and midline velar bulk to contribute the levator eminence and velar extension, which also enhances midline contact in velopharyngeal closure. Salpingopharyngeus muscle occupies salpingopharyngeal fold. It extends from posteroinferior tip of the medial end of the Eustachian tube to posteriorly into the palatopharyngeus at the junction of the velum and lateral pharyngeal wall. The palatopharyngeus extends from velum superiorly to larynx inferiorly and pharyngeal wall posteriorly. It occupies central fifty percent of the velar length. It has two heads lying on nasal and oral side of levator. The palatal head is more developed than nasal. The fibers of the palatopharyngeus thin out and merge with those of levator in paramedian zone. Two heads of palatopharyngeus blend to forms a broad sheet of muscle lateral to the levator. Most of the fibers runs posteriorly forming posterior faucial pillar and inferiorly fuse with the superior constrictor. The palatopharyngeus forms the cleft muscle of veau along with the fibers of the levator and insert along the posterior edge of the hard palate. The palatopharyngeus in conjuction with the antagonistic action of the levator modulates velar position, size and shape to optimize velopheryngeal closure. Along with the superior constrictor, it causes medial displacements of the posterior pharyngeal wall and contributes to the passavant ridge.

Palatoglossus is a slender muscle arises from the transverse muscle fibers of the tongue passes superiorly in the anterior faucial pillar and insert into the muscle of the soft palate. In cleft patients it passes into cleft margin at the posterior edge of the hard palate. Superior constrictor is a quadrangular muscle arises anteriorly from the posterior border of the medial pterygoid plate from the level of the hard palate to the tip of hamulus. This origin continues on a downward and forward slop along the pterygomandibular ligament and muscle sweeps around the pharynx to forms its lateral and posterior wall. It insert posteriorly into the pharyngeal ligament. The superior constrictor causes medial excursion  of the lateral pharyngeal wall by a sphincteric mechanism along with palatopharyngeus. It causes the anterior displacement of posterior pharyngeal wall by fibers that meet across the posterior midline. It is main component of the passavant ridge. Descending palatine artery, a terminal branch of internal maxillary artery gives off several branches to the tonsils and soft palate. It then passes through the posterior palatine foramen, just above the periosteum and proceed forward close to the alveolar margin on each side as the greater palatine artery to the incisive fossa. It sends terminal branch through the incisive foramen to anastomoses  with the terminal branch of the sphenopalatine artery. The sphenopalatine artery is a branch of internal maxillary artery. One of its branches descends to the incisive canal anastomosis with the terminal ascending branch of the posterior palatine artery to form blood supply of the palate. The posterior septal artery arises from the sphenopalatine artery in the roof of the nasal cavity and courses down the groove of the vomer to incisive foramen. The greater palatine artery supplies the oral surface of the hard palate and gives off a few fine branches which perforate the horizontal plate of maxilla to supply the nasal mucosa. It also sends twigs to the gum and palatoglossal arch. The lesser palatine artery suppies about the anterior half of oral surface of the soft palate. The ascending palatine artery, a branch of facial artery, is the largest vessel entering soft palate. It ascends on the lateral side of the superior constrictor muscle to turn downwards and forwards into the soft palate between the tensor and levator palatini. There are two anterior and posterior terminal branches. The vascular supply of the soft palate is not endangered by the operative procedure. In complete bilateral cleft lip and palate, union of superior labial arteries lacking. There is no anastomoses between posterior septal artery with greater palatine artery. Therefore, premaxilla and philtrum derive their blood supply from the posterior septal artery and lateral and terminal branches of the anterior ethmoidal vessels which pass through the columella. The blood supply to the palate enters through the bone and not as in the other parts of the body through periosteum. It is therefore possible at operation to strip the periosteum from its bony attachments without interfering with the blood supply. The hard palate and its mucoperiosteal membrane are supplied by blood from nasopalatine vessels and from the descending palatine arteries. The bony palate has independent blood supply and is thus protected from necrosis following conventional palate surgeries. The sensory branches to the palate are supplied by the maxillary division of the trigeminal nerve. The facial nerve provides secretary and sympathetic fibers to the maxillary division through sphenopalatine ganglion. The greater palatine nerve descends through the greater palatine canal, emerges through the greater palatine foramen and run anteriorly to supply the bony palate and mucous membrane of hard palate. Branches of sphenopalatine nerve emerges from the incisive foramen to the anterior hard palate. The lesser palatine nerve descend through lesser palatine foramen to supply uvula, soft palate and tonsils. The motor supply to the tensor veli palatine is defferent from the other velopharyngeal muscles. The tensor is innervated by the intarnal pterygoid nerve, a branch of the mandibular nerve the third division of trigeminal nerve.

Glossopharyngeal nerve, pharyngeal branch of vagus nerve and accessory nerve supply moter fibers to muscles of pharynx and soft palate except tensor veli palatini muscle. Levator veli palatini. Uvula and superior constrictor muscles are dually innervated by the facial nerve and pharyngeal plexus. Nasal grimacing during phonation in patients with velopharyngeal insufficiency augments the firing of the facial nerve to complement velopharyngeal movements.

## EAR PATHOLOGY

Alt described correlation between ear disease and cleft palate in 1878. Incidence of otitis media[5] is high in cleft palate patients due to abnormalities in Eustachian tube function. Impairment of tubal dilatation due to complex malalignment of paratubal musculature occurs. Chronic obstruction of drainage causes serous otitis media and long-standing effusion leads to hearing loss. Otoscopy, impedance test and audiography are useful in cleft cases. Myringotomy with placement of ventilating tubes remains the mainstay of treatment.[6]

## Presentation

Cleft palate is commonly seen in combination with cleft lip. The alveolar portion of cleft lies between canine and lateral incisor. The lateral incisors are small and dysmorphic on cleft side. There may be delay in eruption or even absence of teeth particularly in operated cases. Unilateral cases have direct communication between nasal passage and oropharynx. The nasal septum is deviated and buckled towards cleft side.

The premaxillary segment containing central and lateral incisor tooth roots is discontinuous from lateral alveolar arch in complete bilateral cleft lip and palate. Locking out of the premaxilla results from collapse of lateral segment inward and lingually. Cleft of secondary palate, known as incomplete cleft palate have variable defect from an opening in the posterior soft palate to cleft extending up to the incisive foramen. Calnan's classic triad of a midline clear zone, a bifid uvula and a palpable notch in the posterior hard palate is present in the submucous cleft palate.[7,8] A distinct midline muscle diastasis is seen with velar muscular contraction. Asymptomatic submucous cleft palate may be closely monitored with serial speech evaluation and audiometry. The Furlow double opposing Z-plasty is an ideal procedure for symptomatic patients. Pharyngeal flaps and sphincter pharyngeoplasty have potential risk of nasal obstruction and sleep apnea.

Pierre Robin had described triad of micrognathia, glossoptosis and respiratory distress. A 60–90% patients with Pierre Robin sequence have cleft palate. Cleft palate defect may vary from small defect in soft palate to V-shaped or more typically U-shaped defect in hard palate. Newborns with Pierre Robin sequence have severe respiratory and feeding difficulties due to posterior displacement of tongue. Initially patients are kept prone and feeding tube are placed for feeding and pushing tongue forward. Nasal airways are useful. Tongue-lip adhesion are effective.

Mandibular distraction osteogenesis has been used in neonates successfully.[9] Tracheostomy is done if all above mentioned procedures fail. Cleft repair is done before decannulation of tracheostomy at age of one year in severe cases. Usually, mandible attains reasonable size in first year of life and cleft palate repair can be performed. Cleft palate have 50% incidence of multiple malformation or syndromes while cleft lip with cleft palate have 30% incidence of syndromic malformation. Van der Woude syndrome is associated with a mutation in the interferon regulatory factor 6 gene and have lower lip sinus tracts and also causes popliteal pterygium syndrome. It is an autosomal dominant syndrome. Syndromic children may have increased incidence of cardiac anomalies. Velocardiofacial syndrome associated with 22q chromosomal delation have characteristic bird like face, soft palate dysfunction, developmental delay and various cardiac conditions.

## Feeding and Swallowing

The palate is barrier between the respiratory tract and alimentary tract. Oral intake has two separate activities: Generation of suction force and swallowing. Lip closes anteriorly and velum seals off pharynx to produce negative intraoral pressure. The primary goal of cleft palate repair is to achieve normal speech. Speech can not be normalized without cleft palate repair. Cleft palate repair separates oropharynx from nasopharynx. Levator veli palatini elevate the palate, create positive pressure in oropharynx for production of sound. Velopharyngeal insufficiency due to noncorrection of cleft palate leads to hypernasal speech often with hoarse quality due to difficulty in directing air flow through the mouth. Victor Veau noted that children who had undergone repair before 12 months have better speech than those who had surgery between 2–4 years of age. Children had worst outcome of surgery, if done after 9 years of age.

Phonological development actually begins early at age of 4–6 months. Some surgeons are suggesting cleft palate repair earlier around 6 months or before for improving feeding but long-term results are lacking. Growing body supports cleft palate repair between 9 and 10 months of age for children with normal development.

Cleft palate repair has been shown to have detrimental effect on maxillary growth.[10] Many patients with repaired cleft palate have transverse maxillary deficiency requiring orthodontic widening of the maxilla once permanent teeth have erupted. Transverse growth of the maxillary arch is narrowed resulting in malocclusion traits of crowding, lateral cross bite and open bite. Maxillary growth inhibition is due to surgical scaring and inherent maxillary under development.

## CLEFT PALATE REPAIR

Under general anesthesia, patient is kept in supine position with neck extension with bolster under the shoulder.

RAE endotracheal tube with throat pack is used. Throat pack is smaller than used in cleft lip repair.

Dingman mouth gag is used. Dingman mouth gag can cause tongue edema if kept for more than two hours. Lidocaine 0.5% and epinephrine 1:200000 are infiltrate into palate maximum up to 1 mL/kg.
Surgery is started after 7–10 minutes of injection.

Cleft palate repair is done with standing surgeon at the child's head. Painting and draping is done bipolar cautery and coblator, if available are used for hemostasis. Incision on each side is kept with surgeon's contralateral hand. Greater palatine neurovascular bundle emerges through the greater palatine foramen at the posterolateral aspect of hard palate. Circumferencial freeing of attachments around the pedicle and gentle stretching of pedicle are important for tension free closure of palate. We prefer 4-0 vicryl for nasal and oral layer closure. Intermittent stitches in nasal layer and horizontal matress stitches are preffered in oral layer.

### von Langenbeck Repair

Bernhard von Langenbeck described simple approximation of the cleft margins with a relaxing incision that began posterior to maxillary tuberosity and followed the posterior portion of the alveolar ridge. Intravelar veloplasty or repair of levator veli palatini is added.[11]
- V-Y Pushback (Veau-Wardill-Kilner) (Fig. 8.3)
- Anterior W-incision is kept.

Bilateral mucoperiosteal flaps based on greater palatine vessels are elevated.

The levator veli palatini muscles are freed from posterior border of the hard palate.

The muscles are repaired across midline with 4-0 vicryl along with nasal layer.

Oral layer is closed in Y-manner to create additional length.

Betadine packs are kept lateraly in raw area (Figs 8.4 to 8.10).

## TWO-FLAP PALATOPLASTY

Large two flaps based on greater palatine vessels are elevated. Intravelar veloplasty is carried out. Suturing is done. This reduces chances of anterior fistula (Figs 8.11 to 8.25).

### Vomer Flaps

Superiorly based vomerine flaps are useful for two layer closure of cleft palate. Vomerine flap is reflected from the nasal septum near cleft margin to close the nasal mucosa of opposite side. Midline incision is kept in bilateral cleft

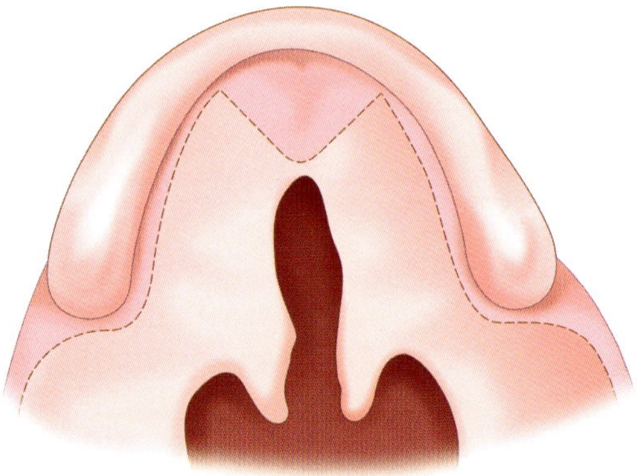

**Fig. 8.3:** V-Y pushback repair. Anterior "W" incision

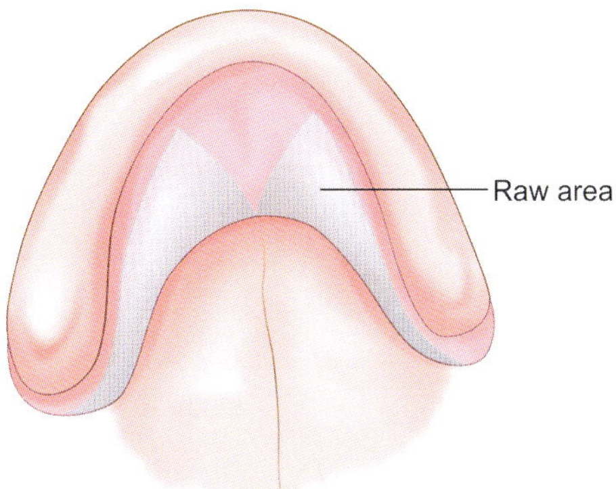



**Fig. 8.4:** At the end of the repair, there are row areas left laterally row areas will heal within 14 days

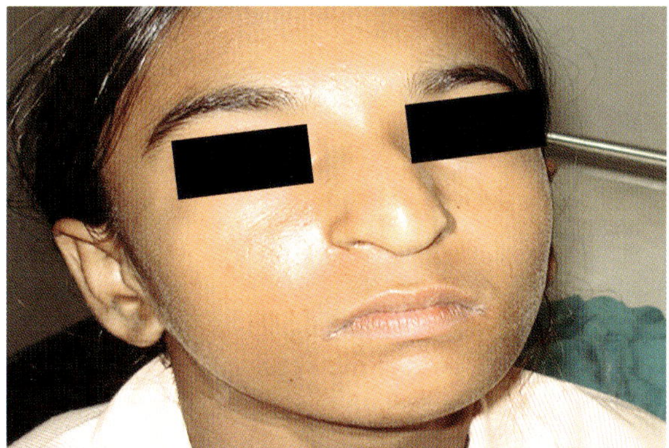

**Fig. 8.5:** Patient with incomplete cleft palate

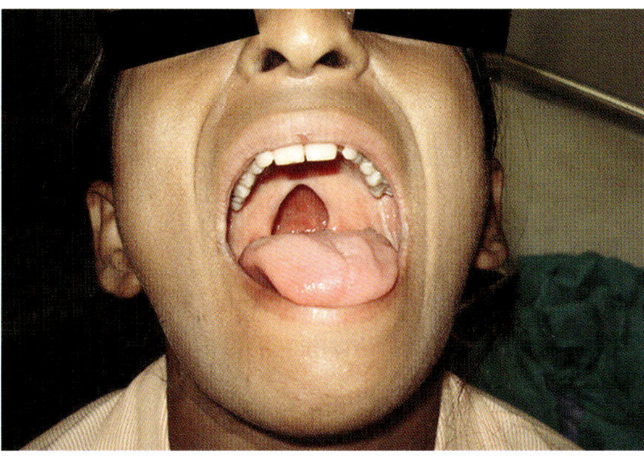

**Fig. 8.6:** Incomplete cleft palate

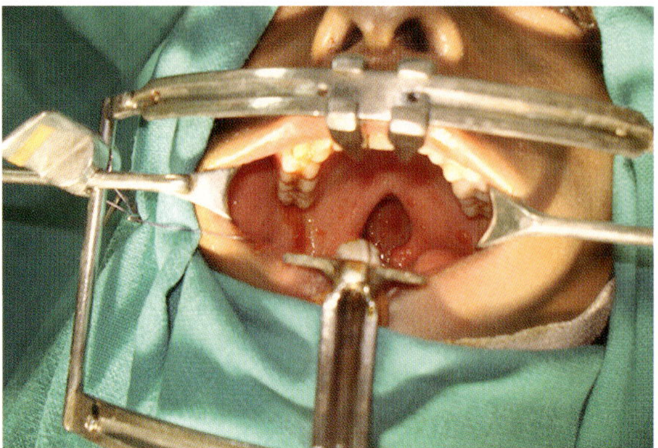

**Fig. 8.7:** Dingman's mouth gag applied (I)

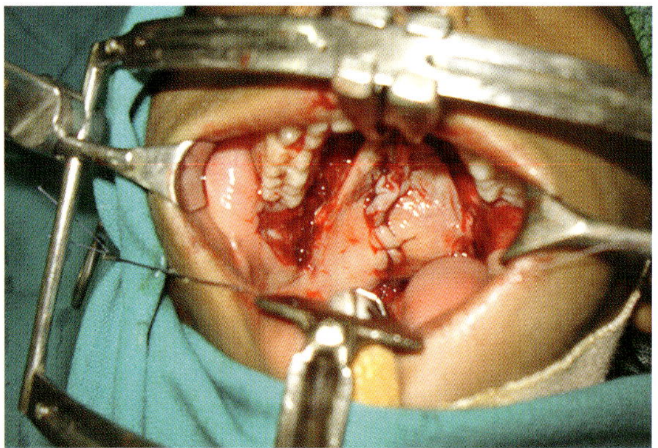

**Fig. 8.8:** Cleft palate repaired with two long flap palatoplasty

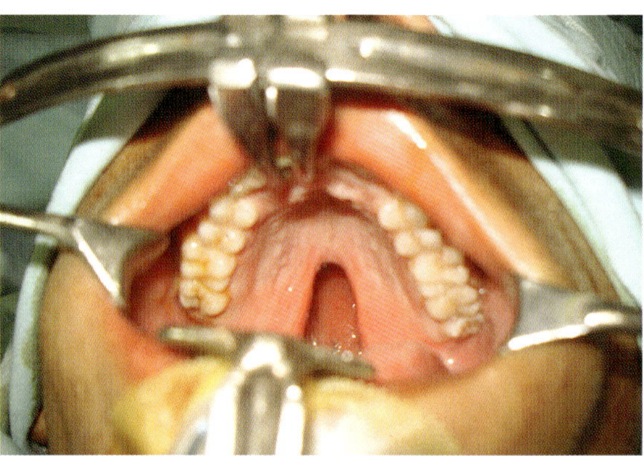

**Fig. 8.9:** Incomplete cleft palate

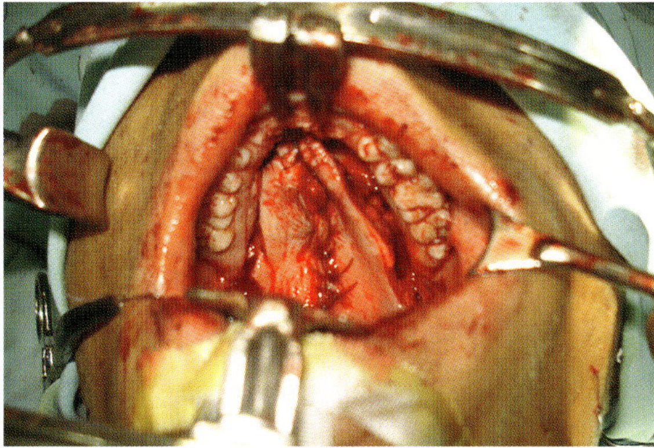

**Fig. 8.10:** Pushback repair palatoplasty

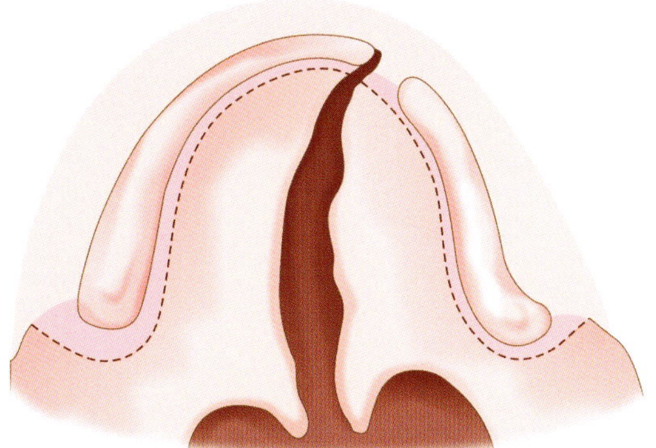

**Fig. 8.11:** Two long flap palatal repair

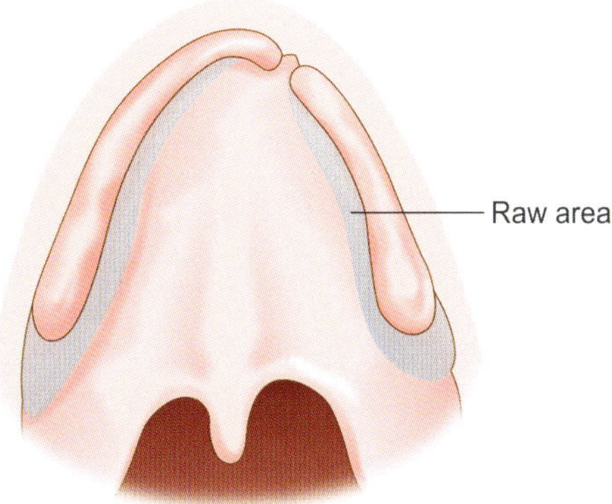


**Fig. 8.12:** Two long flaps reduce chances of anterior fistula

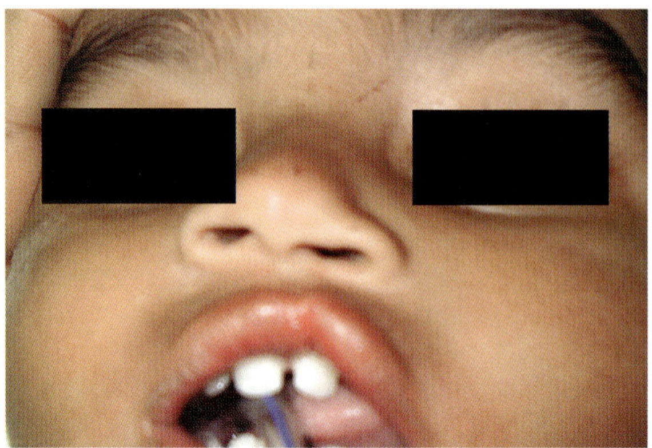

**Fig. 8.13:** Left complete cleft palate (lip operated)

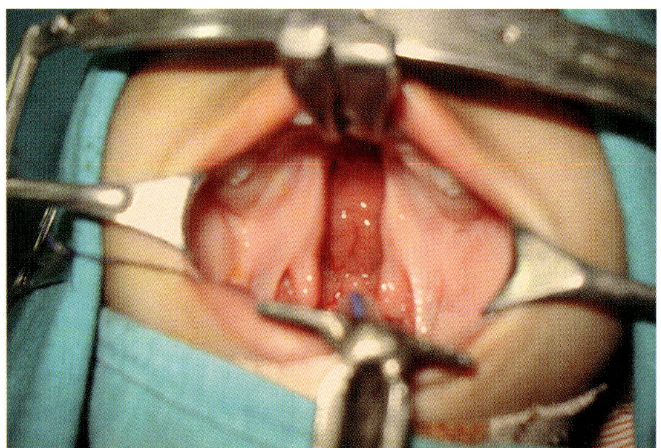

**Fig. 8.14:** Left complete cleft palate

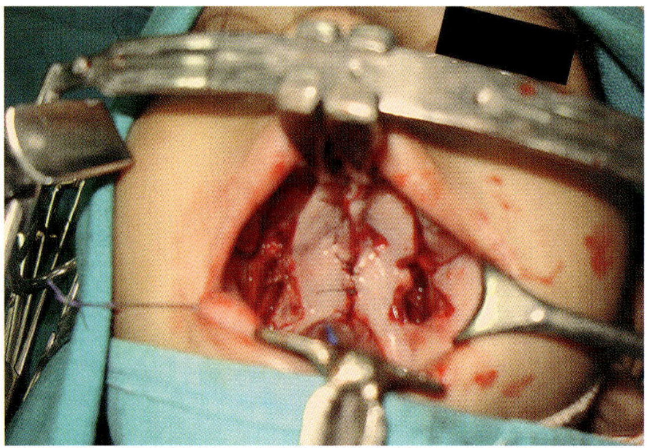

**Fig. 8.15:** Two long flap palatoplasty

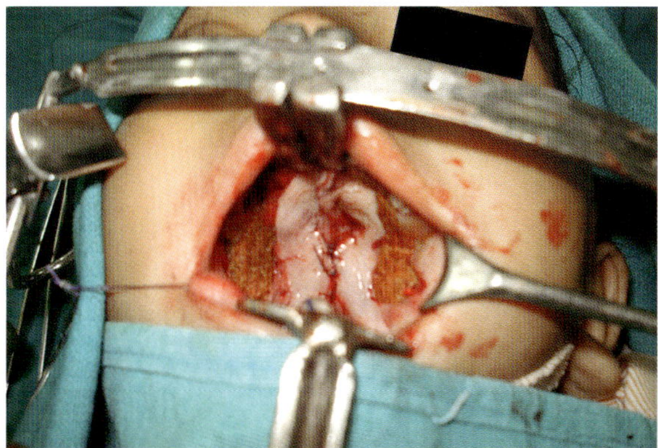

**Fig. 8.16:** Laterally betadine packs were kept for hemostasis

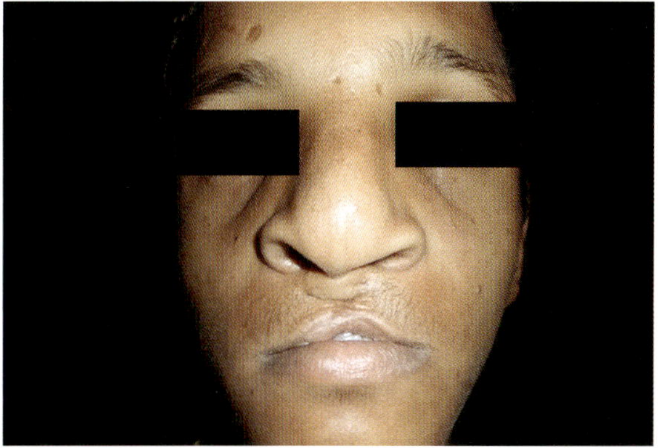

**Fig. 8.17:** Bilateral complete cleft lip with palate (lip operated)

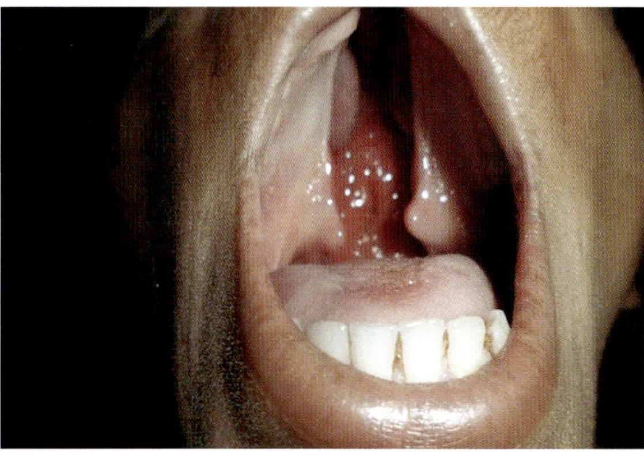

**Fig. 8.18:** Complete cleft palate with wide gap

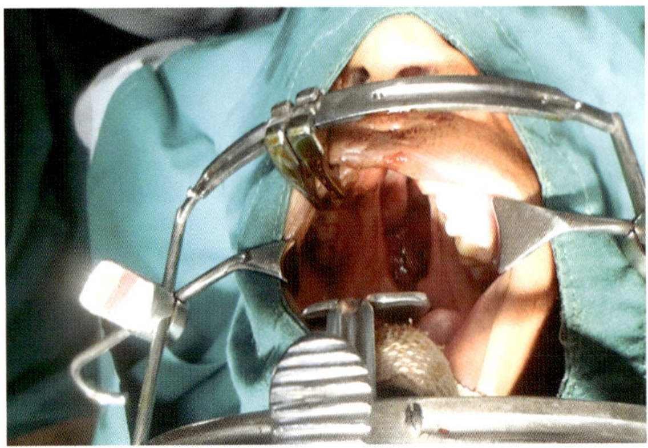

**Fig. 8.19:** Dingman's mouth gag applied (II)

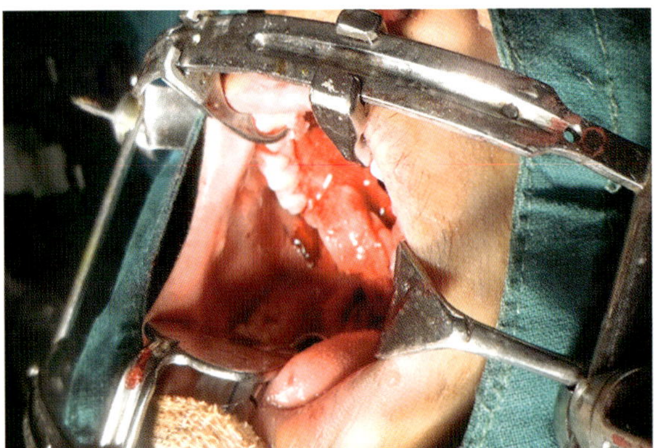

**Fig. 8.20:** Two long flap raised on greater palatine vessels

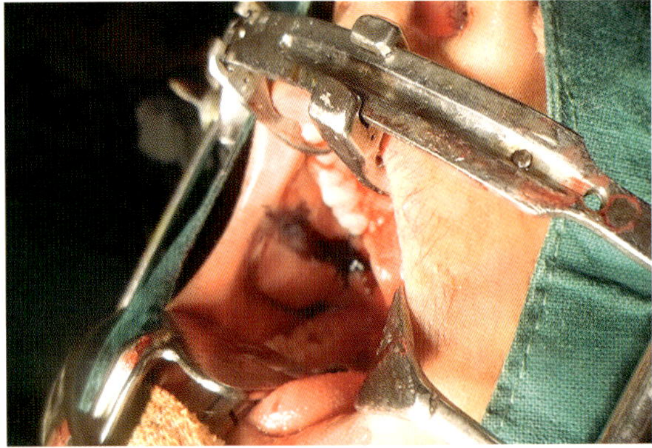

**Fig. 8.21:** Buccal mucosal flap for nasal layer defect planned

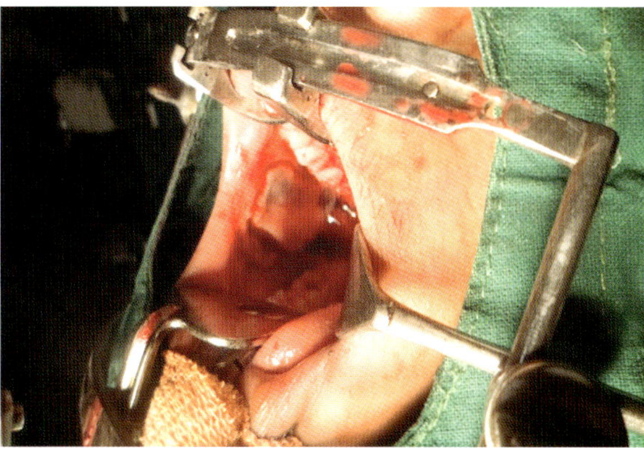

**Fig. 8.22:** Incision kept for island buccal mucosal flap

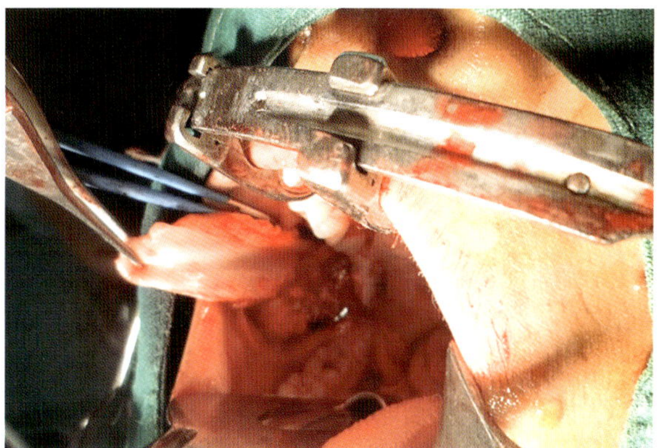

**Fig. 8.23:** Buccal flap was raised

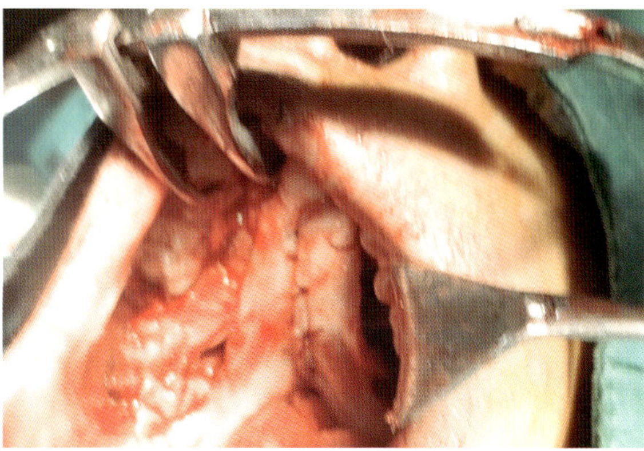

**Fig. 8.24:** Final closure done

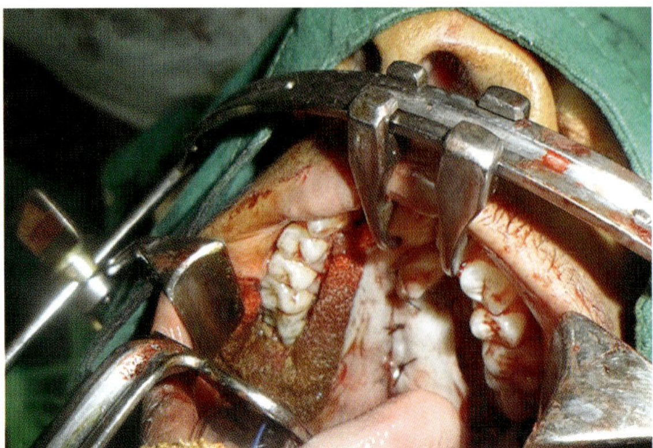

**Fig. 8.25:** Betadine packs were kept laterally and over bucal defect for hemostasis

palate. Two flaps are reflected on both sides and nasal layer are closed. It has low fistula rate with less effect on maxillary growth.

## Intravelar Veloplasty

Victor Veau was first to describe midline reapproximation of the levator veli palatini muscles. Braithwaite described extensive muscle dissection for posterior repositioning and tension-free approximation. He described careful freeing of levator muscles from posterior edge of the hard palate. Cutting[2] described radical levator transposition with extensive dissection of muscle from both nasal and oral layer. Somerland used microscope for dissection of muscle. Tensor veli palatini is released just medial to hamulus and levator muscle are overlapped in midline.[2] Furlow double opposing Z-plasty has excellent overlapping of levator muscle and so excellent speech outcome in early evaluation. Cutting and Sommerland described re-repair of levator muscle in velopharyngeal insufficiency.

## Furlow Double Opposing Z-plasty[12]

Furlow described double opposing Z-plasty for cleft palate repair in 1980. The oral flap is posteriorly based on left side with the levator muscle. The right side flap is anteriorly based and above muscle. The reverse pattern is planned on nasal side. This repair provides complete nasal and oral closure with levator sling. This technique ignores musculus uvulae muscle. Furlow described use of relaxing incision for closure when necessary. Buccal mucosal flap may be useful along with Z-plasty for nasal and oral layer closure in wide clefts (Figs 8.26 to 8.28).

Schweckendiek and Doz[13] described repair of the soft palate at the same time as the cleft lip repair around 4–5 months of age. The hard palate was obturated and was repaired at age of 4–5 years.[3] Hard palate cleft narrows during the time between the procedure requiring less dissection and thus reducing chances of maxillary growth disturbances. Numerous studies have shown significant poor speech result from these two-stage procedures.

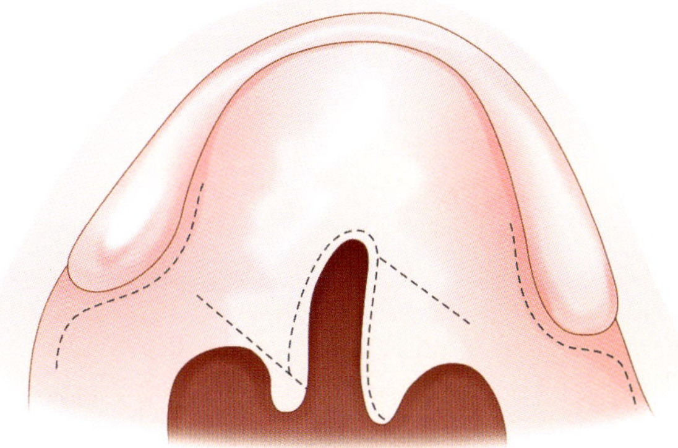

**Fig. 8.26:** Furlow double opposing Z-plasty

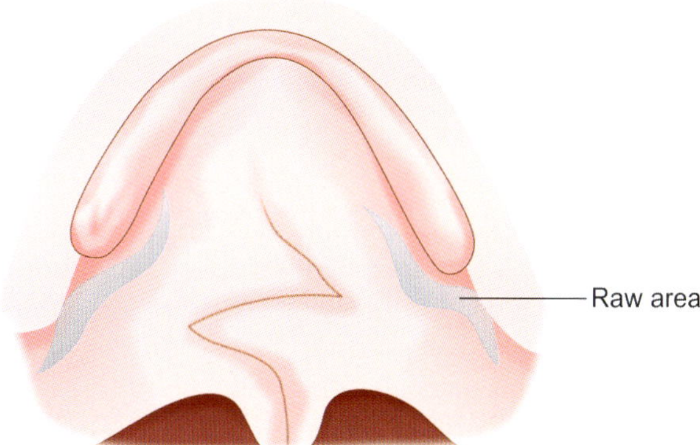



**Fig. 8.27:** Two relaxing incisions laterally helps closure

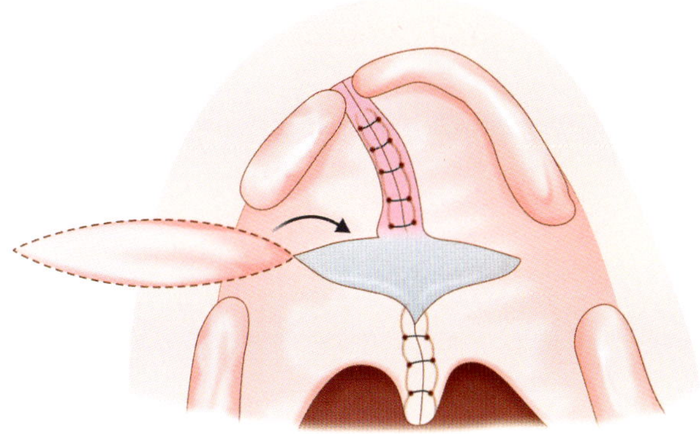

**Fig. 8.28:** Buccal mucosal flap

## POSTOPERATIVE CARE

- Patients are kept nil orally for 4 hours.
- Analgesics ibuprofen 10 mg/kg will usually give adequate pain relief.
- Watch for bleeding, hypoxia particularly in Pierre Robin syndrome cases.
- Lateral position, thread for holding tongue, nasal trumpets are useful.
- Application of ice pack to posterior neck area is useful to stop postoperative bleeding.
- Postoperative feeding is limited to liquids for 14 days to prevent lodging material in raw area left open at end of procedure laterally.

## OUTCOMES OF CLEFT PALATE REPAIR[10]

### Fistulae[14]

Palatal fistula leads to persistant nasal air loss and nasal regurgitation of fluids. Fistula is more common in wide cleft palate and often after two flap surgery than Furlow Z-plasty. Early closure of cleft palate fistula after 3 months of first surgery is recommended particularly with large mucoperiosteal flap or with Von Langenbeck flaps. Palatal plate may aid in obturating a fistula if there is delay in surgery (Figs 8.29 to 8.42).

### Speech Outcome

Normal speech is primary goal of palatoplasty. With early surgery before 1 year of age, good surgical repair with intravelar veloplasty and good postoperative care we can achieve 85–90% good speech result.

The results are better in nonsyndromic than syndromic patients, unilateral cleft then bilateral cleft and narrower than wider clefts.

### Maxillary Growth

Normal maxillary growth is the secondary goal of palatoplasty. We should avoid large raw area on hard palate to minimize scar tissue. Fistula formation requires

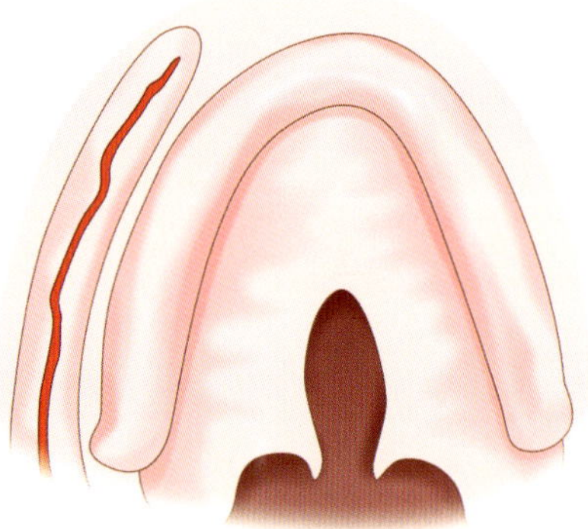

**Fig. 8.29:** Facial artery myomucosal flap

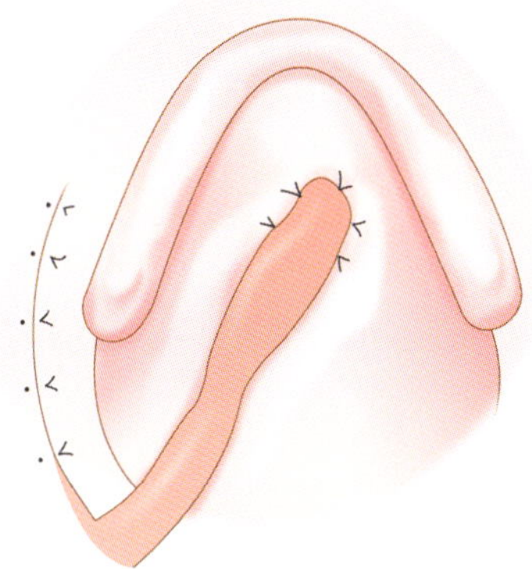

**Fig. 8.30:** Donor site of flap closed primarily

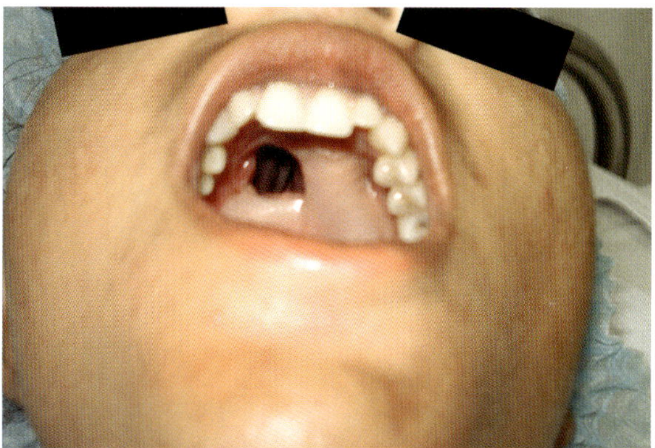

**Fig. 8.31:** Large palatal fistula

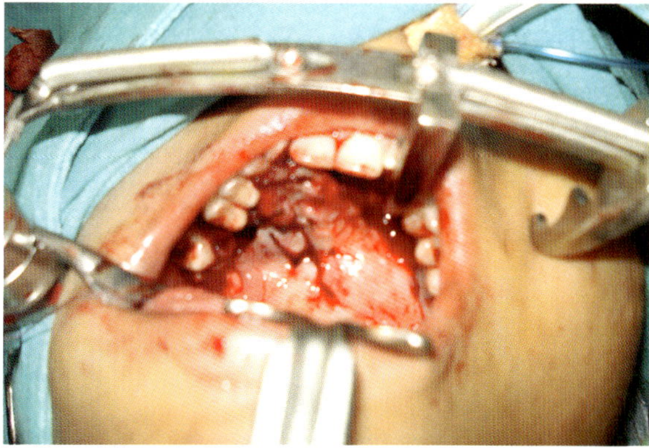

**Fig. 8.32:** Fistula was closed with local palatal flaps

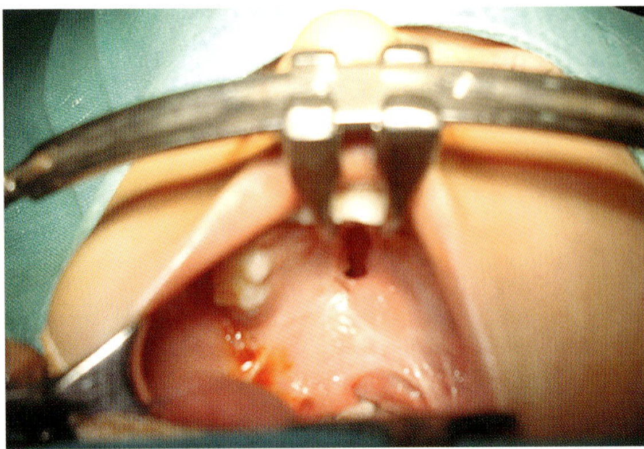

**Fig. 8.33:** Patient with anterior palatal fistula

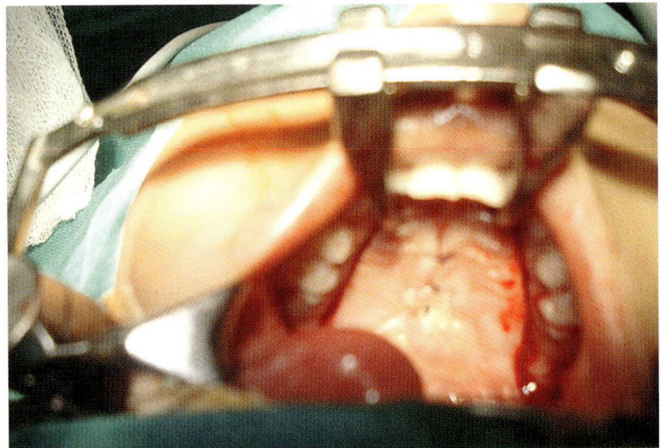

**Fig. 8.34:** Fistula was closed with local palatal flaps

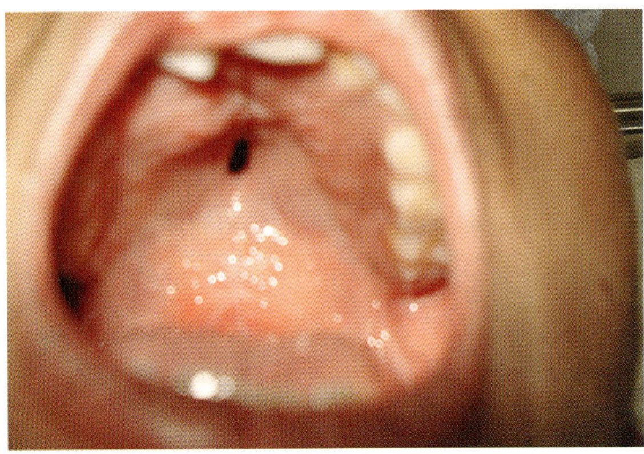

**Fig. 8.35:** Small palatal fistula

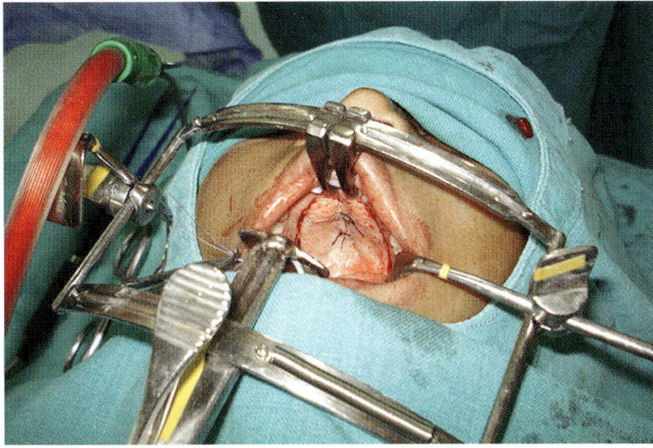

**Fig. 8.36:** Palatal fistula closed with local palatal flap

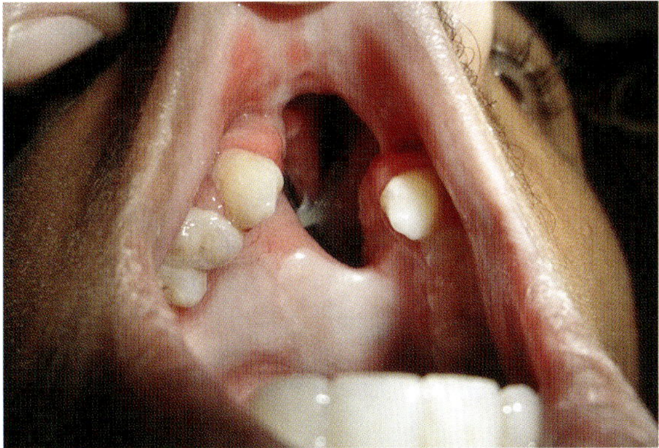

**Fig. 8.37:** Large anterior palatal fistula and alveolar fistula

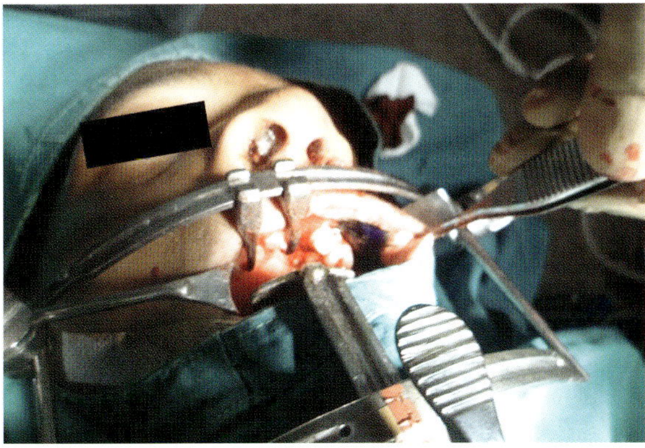

**Fig. 8.38:** Buccal mucosal flap was planned

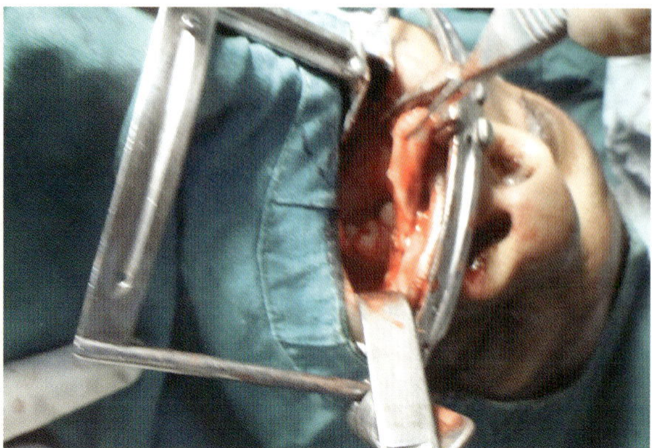

**Fig. 8.39:** Buccal mucosal flap was raised

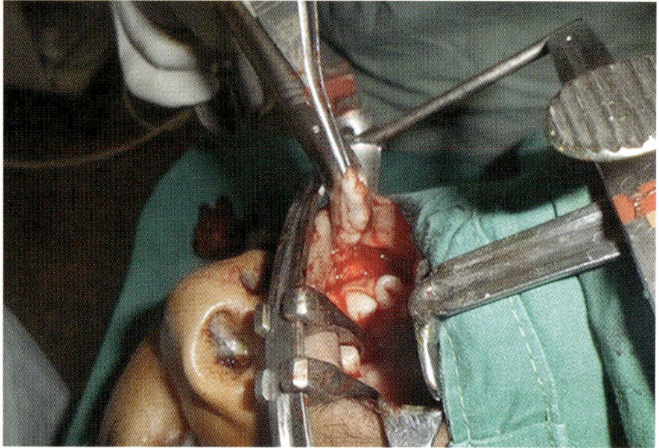

**Fig. 8.40:** Island buccal mucosal flap is brought over anterior part of palate

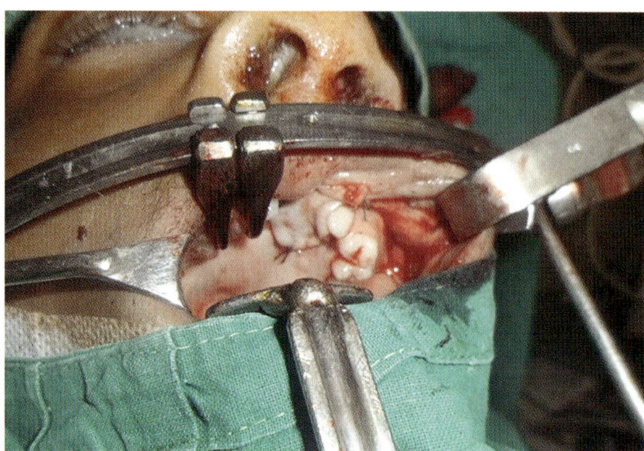

**Fig. 8.41:** Inset completed

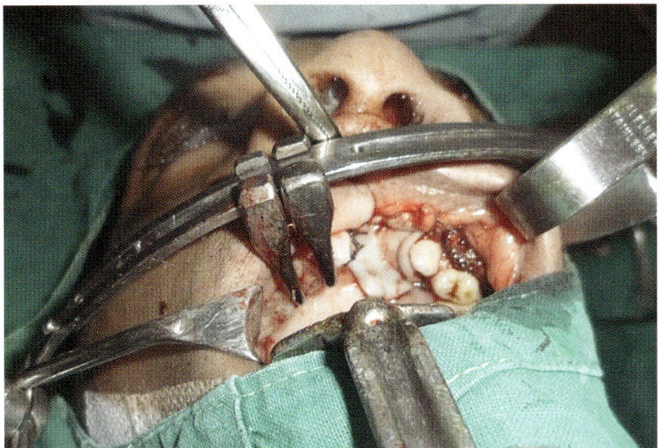

**Fig. 8.42:** Raw area of buccal mucosal flap was kept open for secondary healing

additional procedure for closure will increase scar tissue and decreases maxillary growth. Maxillary hypoplasia is more common in syndromic cleft palate requiring maxillary advancement procedure at puberty.

## REFERENCES


1. Kreins OB. Anatomy of the velopharyngeal area in cleft palate. Clin Plast Surg. 1975;2:261.
2. Cutting C, Rosenbaum J, Rovati L. The technique of muscle repair in soft palate. Operative Techniques Plastic Surgery. 1995;2:215-22.
3. Cosman B, Falk AS. Delayed hard palate repair and speech deficiencies: a cautionary report. Cleft Palate J. 1980;17:2733.
4. Fara M. The musculature of cleft lip and palate. In McCarthy JG, (Ed). Plastic Surgery Philadelphia: WB Saunders. 1991:2598-626.
5. Dhilon RS. The middle ear in cleft palate children pre and post palatal closure. J R Soc Med. 1988;81:710-13.
6. Paradise JL. Middle ear problems associated with cleft palate. An internationally oriented review. Cleft palate J. 1975;12:1722.
7. Chen PK, Wu J, Hung KF, et al. Surgical correction of submucous cleft palate with furlow palatoplasty. Plast Reconstr Surg. 1996;97:1136-46.
8. Kaplan EN. The occult submucous cleft palate. Cleft palate J. 1975;12:356-68.
9. Denny AD, Talisman R, Hanson PR, et al. Mandibular distraction osteogenesis in very young patients to correct airway obstruction. Plast Reconstr Surg. 2001;108:302-11.
10. Bardach J, Morris HL, Olin WH. Late results of primary veloplasty: the Marburg Project. Plast Reconstr Surg. 1984;73(2):207-18.
11. Pensler JM, Baurer BS. Levator repositioning and palatal lengthening for submucous clefts. Plast Reconstr Surg. 1988;82:765-9.
12. Furlow Jr LT. Cleft palate repair by double opposing Z-plasty. Plast Reconstr Surg. 1986;78:724.
13. Sehweckendiek W, Doz P. Primary veloplasty: long-term results without maxillary deformity—a 25 years report. Cleft palate J. 1978;15:268.
14. Emory Jr RE, Clay RP, Bite U, et al. Fistula formation and repair after palatal closure: an institutional perspective. Plast Reconstr Surg. 1997;99:1535-8.

# CHAPTER 9

# Management of Velopharyngeal Dysfunction

Velopharyngeal insufficiency is due to inability to achieve complete closure of velopharyngeal apparatus during speech. The velopharyngeal apparatus includes soft palate and pharyngeal structures that regulate airflow from lungs and larynx through mouth for oral sounds and through the nose for nasal sounds. Velopharyngeal dysfunction[1] may be due to structural defect, neuromotor pathologies or velopharyngeal mislearning. Plastic surgeons are involved in velopharyngeal dysfunction due to clefting of secondary palate. There is often lack of sufficient soft palate tissue, scar tissue or fistula of hard palate or soft palate.

## ASSESSMENT OF VELOPHARYNGEAL FUNCTION

1. **Perceptual speech evaluation:** Hypernasality means the perception of inordinate nasal resonance during the production of vowels, nasal emission means the escape of nasal air associated with the production of consonants that require high oral pressure, nasal substitution, compensatory articulation and sibilant distortion means incorrect tongue placement often due to malocclusion are noted in patients with cleft.

2. **Pressure flow measurements:** The pressure flow technique allows quantitative measurement of pressure, airflow and timing variable associated with velopharyngeal closure.

3. **Nasopharyngeal endoscopy:** Video nasopharyngeal endoscopy[2] permits direct observation of the velopharyngeal apparatus during speech.[2,3] Movement of soft palate posterior pharynx and lateral pharyngeal wall are seen through small nasopharyngoscope (Figs 9.1 to 9.5).[4]

4. **Cinefluoroscopy:** Cinefluoroscopy of the velopharynx can provide dynamic visualization of the velopharynx. Resting and phonating lateral cephalometric audiographs can give fair idea of velopharyngeal insufficiency.

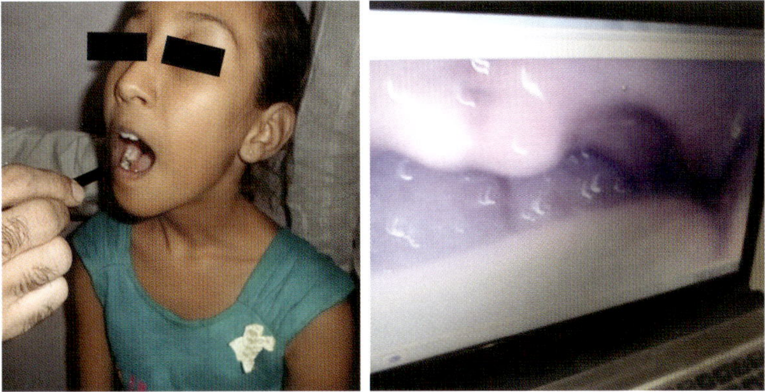

**Fig. 9.1:** Video endoscopy of a patient with submucuos cleft palate

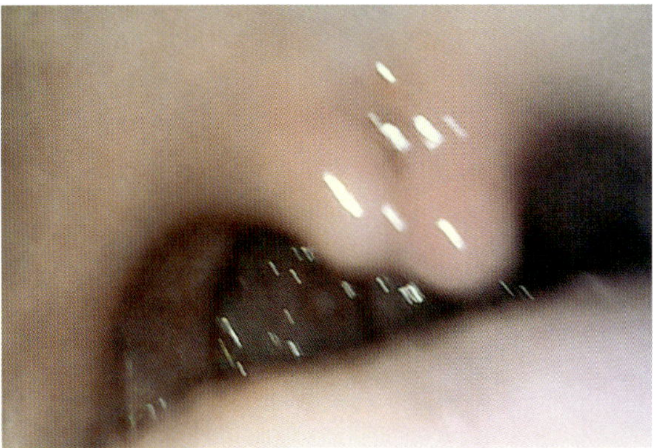

**Fig. 9.2:** Video endoscopy for submucous cleft palate

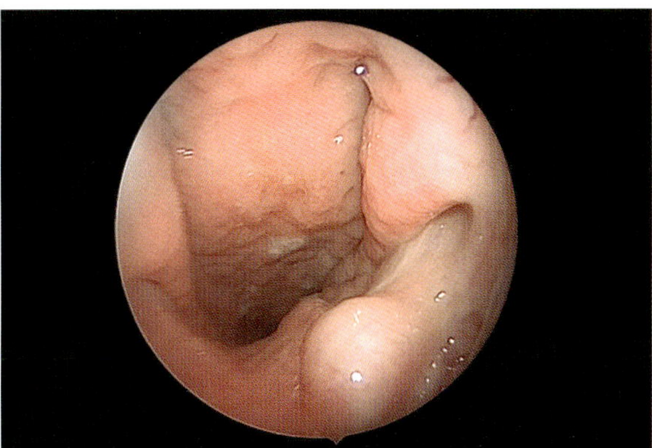

**Fig. 9.3:** Nasoendoscopy showing velopharyngeal insufficiency
*Source:* Dr Yash Pandya

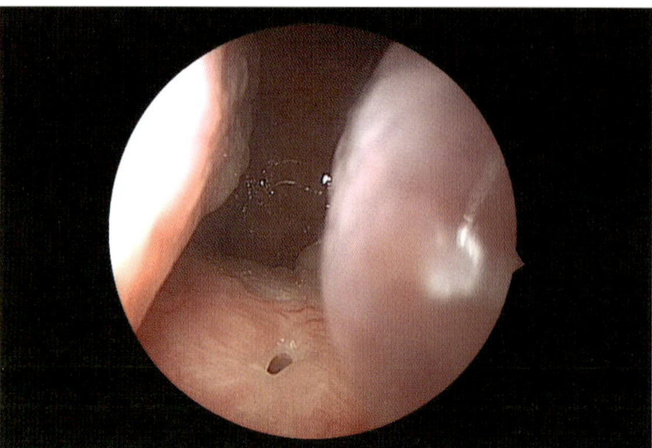

**Fig. 9.4:** Nasoendoscopy showing palatal fistula from nasal side

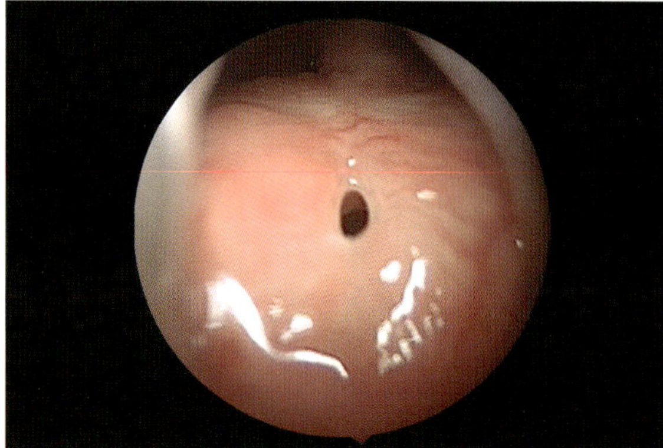

**Fig. 9.5:** Palatal fistula seen in nasoendoscopy

Levator muscle[5] repositioning with palatal lengthening with or without use of buccal mucosal flap gives good results of surgery particularly done before 2 years of age.

Furlow palatoplasty with or without use of buccal mucosal flap have excellent speech outcome, particularly if velopharyngeal gap is less than 8 mm.[6-9]

## POSTERIOR PHARYNGEAL FLAP[10-12]

Schoenborn described inferiorly based posterior pharyngeal flap in 1886. Padgett popularized the posterior pharyngeal flap in the United States used superiorly based flap. Hogan introduced concept of lateral port control in superiorly based pharyngeal flap and suggested 4 mm size of port on both sides of flap (Figs 9.6 to 9.25).

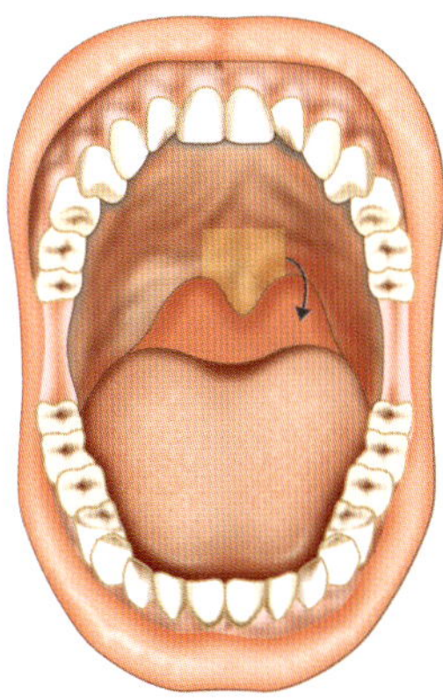

**Fig. 9.6:** Inferiorly based posterior pharyngeal flap

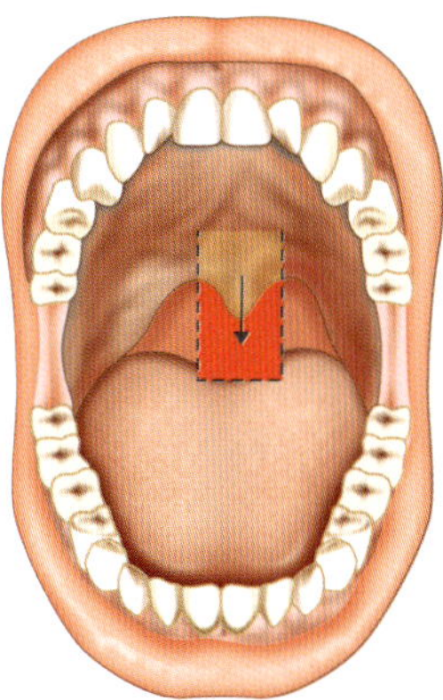

**Fig. 9.7:** Superiorly based posterior pharyngeal flap

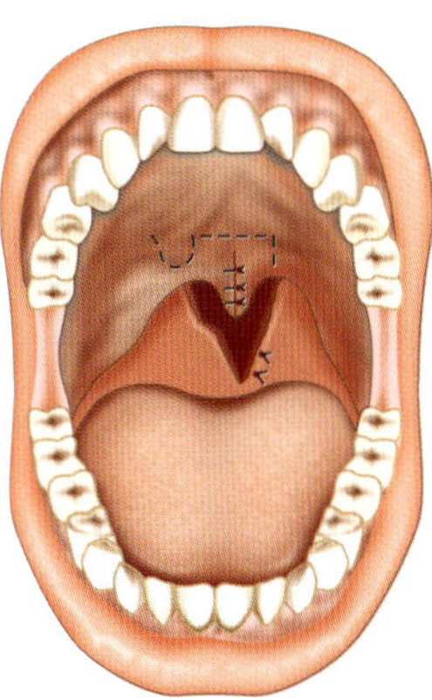

**Fig. 9.8:** Inset of posterior pharyngeal flap and closure of soft palate and uvula completed. Defect of posterior pharyngeal flap is closed primarily

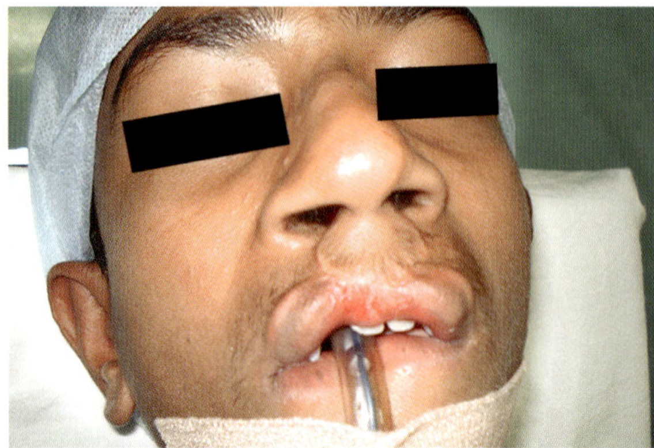

**Fig. 9.9:** Bilateral complete cleft lip with palate (operated)

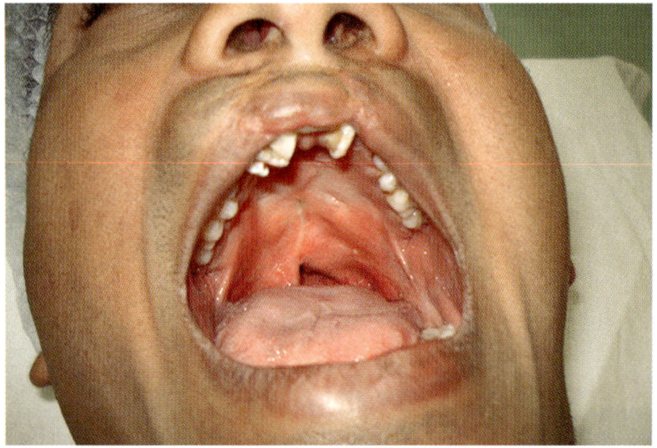

**Fig. 9.10:** Patient had velopharyngeal insufficiency

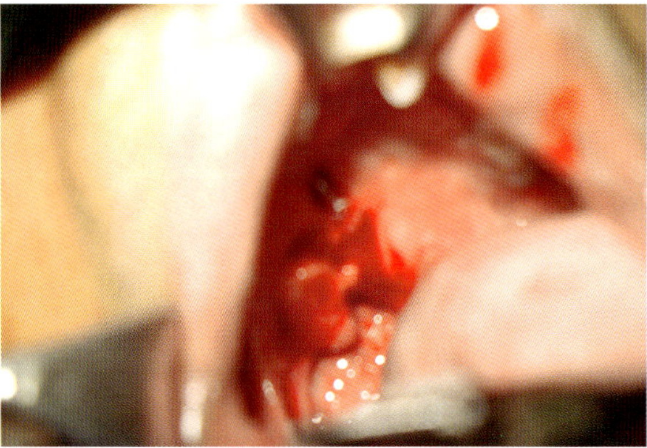

**Fig. 9.11:** U-shaped posteriorly based flap of soft palate is raised

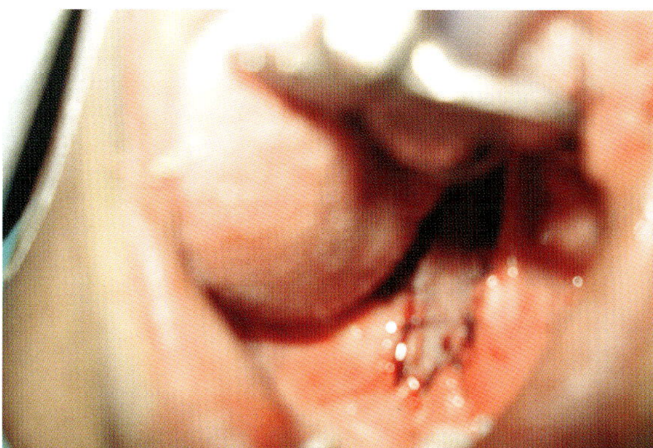

**Fig. 9.12:** Inferiorly based posterior pharyngeal flap

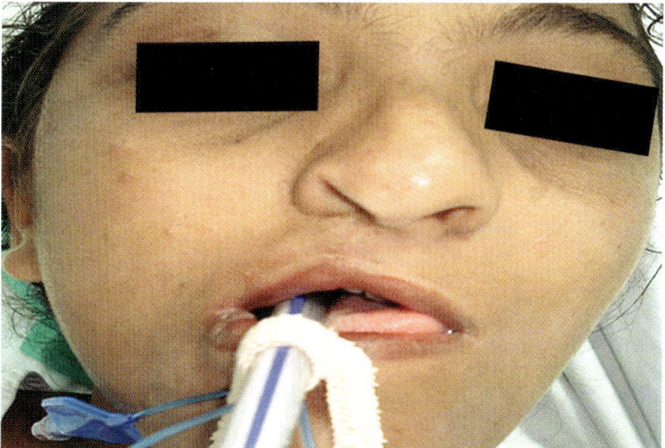

**Fig. 9.13:** Right complete cleft lip with palate (operated)

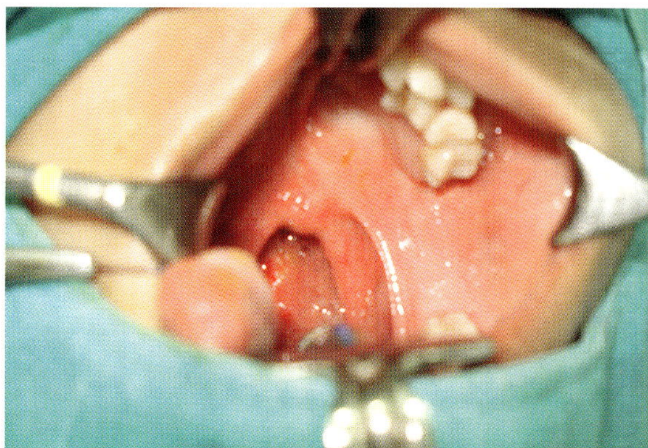

**Fig. 9.14:** Velopharyngeal insufficiency

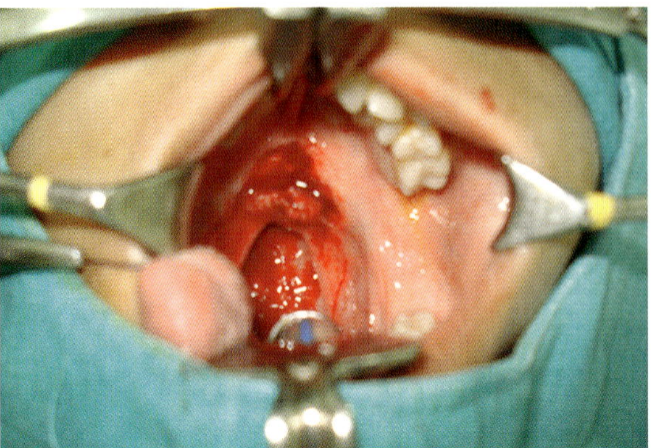

**Fig. 9.15:** Posteriorly based flap raised from soft palate

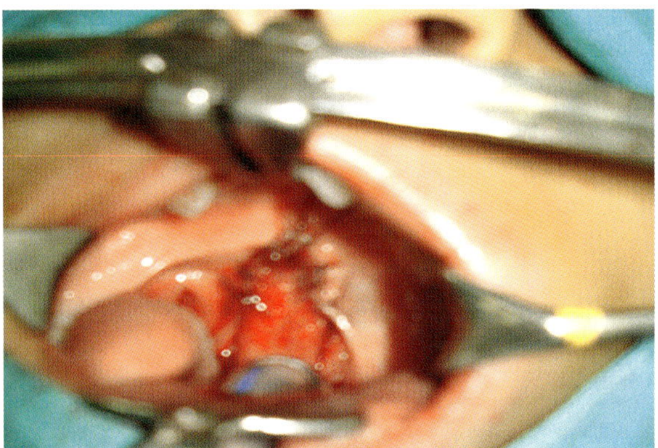

**Fig. 9.16:** Inferiorly based posterior pharyngeal flap sutured to oral layer of soft palate

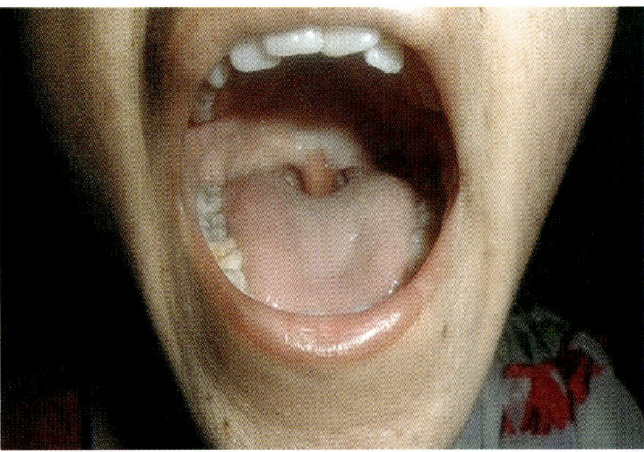

**Fig. 9.17:** Inferiorly based posterior pharyngeal flap after two years of surgery

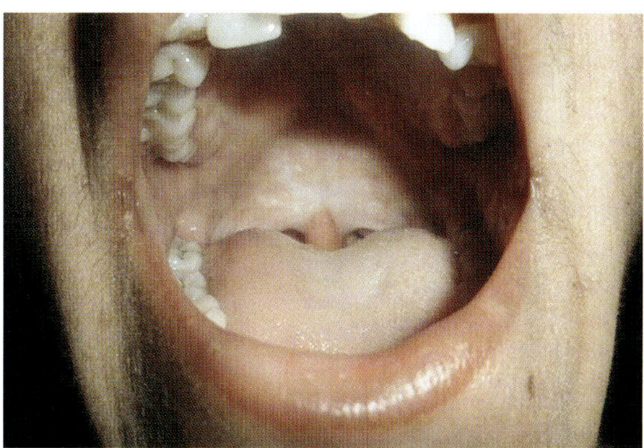

**Fig. 9.18:** Inferiorly based posterior pharyngeal flap is easier to perform

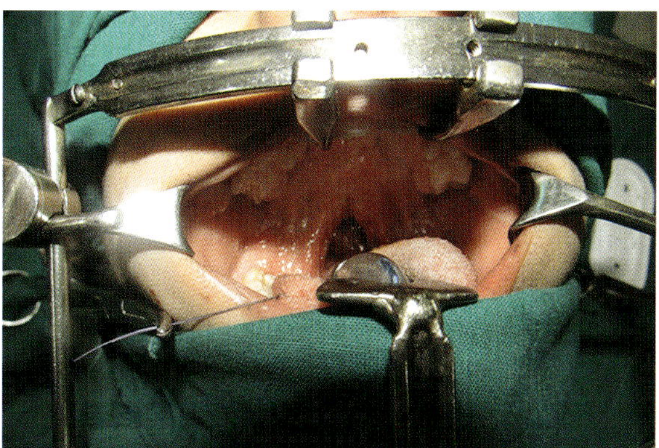

**Fig. 9.19:** Velopharyngeal insufficiency

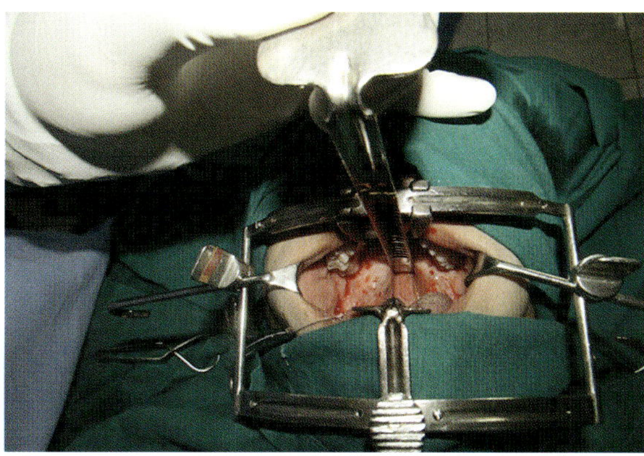

**Fig. 9.20:** Posterior pharyngeal wall is seen

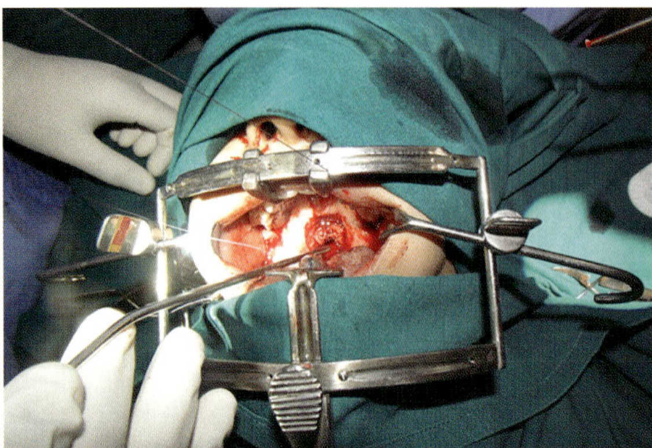

**Fig. 9.21:** U-shaped posteriorly based flap raised from soft palate

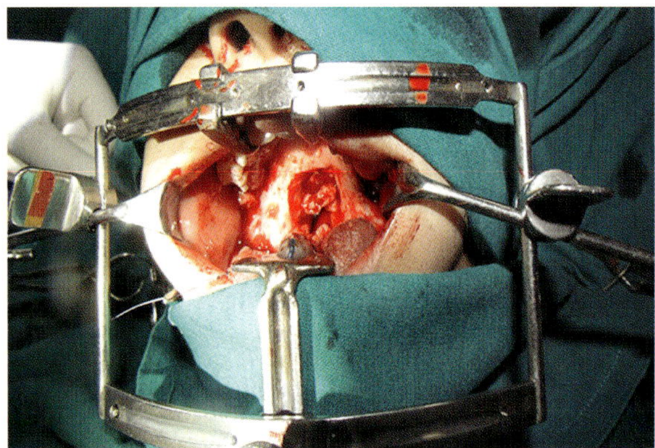

**Fig. 9.22:** Resultant row area is seen over soft palate

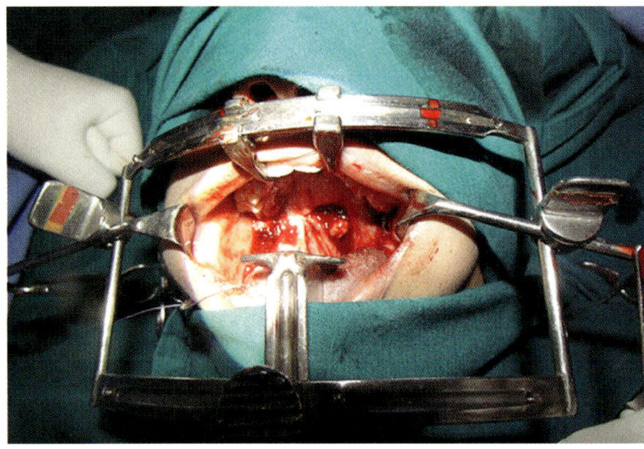

**Fig. 9.23:** Inferiorly posterior pharyngeal flap is raised and inset is given over soft palate

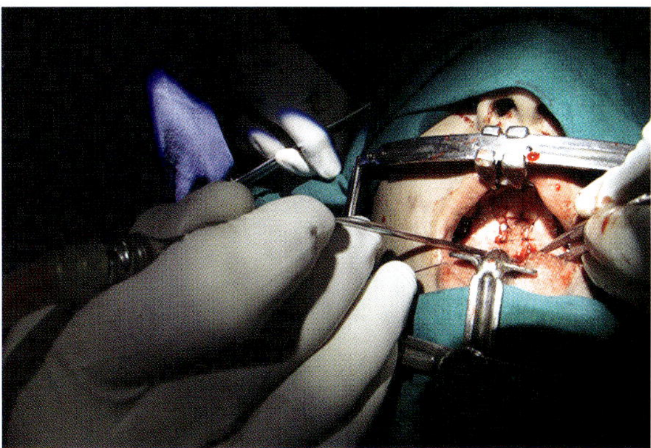

**Fig. 9.24:** In setting of inferior posterior pharyngeal flap is completed

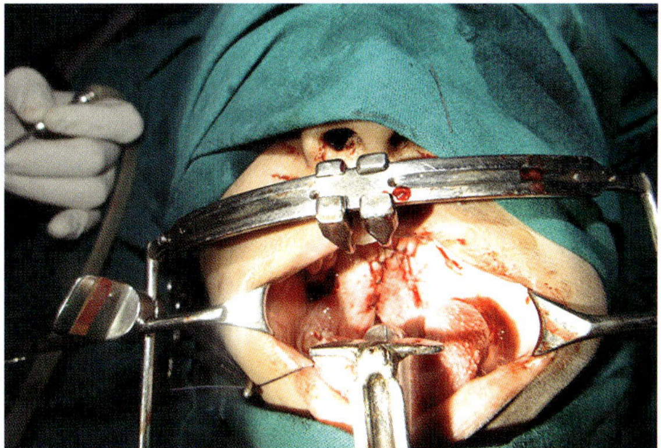

**Fig. 9.25:** Inset of flap: completed with 4-0 vicryl

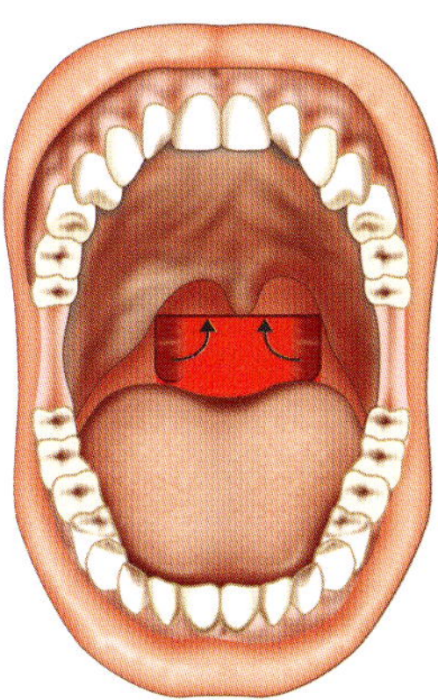

**Fig. 9.26:** Sphincter pharyngoplasty

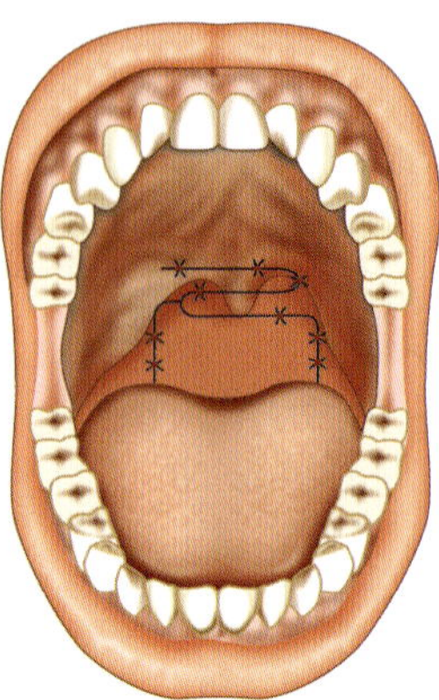

**Fig. 9.27:** Sphincter pharyngoplasty completed

Shprintzen et al. introduced concept of tailor made pharyngeal flap and proposed that the width of the flap should be determined by the amount of lateral pharyngeal wall motion. Length of hospital stay, complications, speech outcome and hearing results were same in superiorly based and inferiorly based posterior pharyngeal flap. Hynes and Orticochea[13-17] described sphincter pharyngoplasty (Figs 9.26 and 9.27). Pharyngoplasty showed improvement in hypernasality and decreased nasal emission. Pharyngoplasty has complications like snoring, swallowing problems, nasal obstruction and difficulty in blowing nose.[18]

Augmentation of posterior pharyngeal wall with fat, fascia, fascia lata[19,20] or with alloplastic[21-24] material like Silicone, Teflon and proplast have been recommended with limited success. There are all chances of spontaneous absorption in autologous tissue and infection and extrusion in alloplastic material.

## REFERENCES


1. Passavant G. Concerning the improvement in speech after operation on the palate. Arch Klin Chir. 1879;23:771-80.
2. Croft CB, Shprintzen RJ, Rakoff SJ. Patterns of velopharyngeal valving in normal and cleft palate subjects: A multi-view videofluroscopic and nasoendoscopic study. Laryngoscope. 1981;91:265-71.
3. Golding-Kushner KJ. Standardization for the reporting of nasopharyngoscopy and multiview videofluoroscopy: A report from an International Working Group. Cleft Palate Craniofac J. 1990;27:337-48.
4. Ysunza A, Pamlona M, Fernat T, et al. Videonasopharyngoscopy as an instrument for visual biofeedback during speech in cleft palate patients. Int J Pediatr Otorhinolaryngol. 1997;24:45-54.
5. Ha S, Krehn DP, Cohen M, et al. Magnetic resonance imaging of the levator veli palatini muscle in speakers with repaired cleft palate. Cleft Palate Cranioface J. 2007;44:494-505.

6. Chen PK, Wu JT, Chen YR, et al. Correction of secondary velopharyngeal insufficiency in cleft palate patients with the Furlow Palatoplasty. Plast Reconstr Surg. 1994;94:933-41.

7. Furlow LT. Cleft palate repair: Preliminary report on lengthening and muscle transposition by Z-plasty. Southeastern Society of Plastic and Reconstructive Surgeons. 1978. Boca Raton, FL.

8. Hundson DA, Grobbelaar AO, Fernandes DB, et al. Treatment of velopharyngeal incompetence by the Furlow Z-plasty. Ann Plast Surg. 1995;34:23-6.

9. Liao YF, Noordhoff MS, huang CS, et al. Comparison of obstructive sleep apnoea following Furlow palatoplasty or pharyngeal flap for velopharyngeal insufficiency. Cleft Palate Craniofac. J. 2004;41:152-6.

10. Cable BB, Canady JW, Karnell MP, et al. Pharyngeal flap surgery: long term outcomes at the University of Iowa. Plast Reconstr Surg. 2004;113:475-8.

11. Sullivan SR, Marinan EM, Mulliken JB. Pharyngeal flap outcomes in nonsyndromic children with repaired cleft palate and velopharyngeal insufficiency. Plast Reconstr Surg. 2010;125:290-8.

12. Ysunza A, Pamplona C, Ramirez E, et al. Velopharyngeal surgery: a prospective randomized study of pharyngeal flaps and sphincter pharyngoplasties. Plast Reconstr Surg. 2002;110:1401-7.

13. Hynes W. Pharyngoplasty by muscle transplantation. Br J Plast Surg. 1950;3:128-35.

14. Hynes W. The results of pharyngoplasty by muscle transplantation in failed cleft palate cases, with special reference to the influence of the pharynx on voice production. Ann R Coll Surg Engl. 1953;13:17-35.

15. Hynes W. Observation on pharyngoplasty. Br J Plast Surg. 1967;20:244-56.

16. Jackson IT, Silverton JS. The sphincter pharyngoplasty as a secondary procedure in cleft palates. Plast Reconstr Surg. 1977;59:518-24.

17. Orticochra M. Construction of a dynamic muscle splincter in cleft palates. Plast Reconstr Surg. 1968;41:323-7.

18. Kuehn DI, Imrey PB, Tomes L, et al. Efficacy of continuous positive airway pressure for treatment of hypernasality. Cleft Palate Craniofac J. 2002;39:267-76.

19. Denny AD, Marks SM, Oriff- Carneo's. Correction of velopharyngeal insufficiency by pharyngeal augmentation using autologous cartilage: A preliminary report. Cleft Palate Craniofac J. 1993;30:46-54.

20. Leuchter I, Schweizer V, Hohlfeld J, et al. Treatment of velopharyngeal insufficiency by autologous fat injection. Euro Arch Otorhinolaryngol. 2010;267:977-83.

21. Blocksma R. Correction of velopharyngeal insufficiency by silastic pharyngeal implant. Plast Reconstr Surg. 1963;31:268-74.

22. Eckstein H. Demonstration of paraffin prosthesis in defects of the face and palate. Dermatology. 1904;11:772-8.

23. Furlow FT, Williams WN, Eisenbach CR, et al. A long term study on treating velopharyngeal insufficiency by Teflon injection. Cleft Palate J. 1982;19:47-56.

24. Lewy R. Teflon injection in correction of velopharyngeal insufficiency. Ann Otos rhinol Laryngol. 1965;74:874.

# CHAPTER 10

# Alveolar Cleft

## INTRODUCTION

The alveolar cleft is more than a linear gap in alveolar arch, gap increase in size from incisal to apical region. The lateral piriform rim is hypoplastic. The maxillary nasal crest is deviated away from the cleft.[1,2] The nasolabial fistula lies high up in the labial sulcus and oronasal fistula extends from incisive foramen to the alveolar process.

The aim of the alveolar bone grafting is to provide a stable supporting environment for eruption of the permanent canine, it stabilize premaxilla in bilateral cleft cases, and provide better support to the base of nose. It bridges hole in alveolar ridge.

Permanent lateral incisor may be absent or may be extracted to create space for the permanent canine to migrate and erupt through newly grafted area.

Gingivoperiosteoplasty is done at the same time as the primary lip repair if alveolar anatomy and presurgical molding outcome are favorable. The gingivoperiosteoplasty is performed after dissection and before repair of the lip elements. The nasal floor closure separates the nasal from oral cavity back to the incisive foramen. The roof of the gingivoperiosteoplasty is the repair of nasal floor from the nasal sill back to the incisive foramen, and floor of the gingivoperiosteoplasty is created by flaps from the oral edges of alveolar cleft. All infants will not be candidates for gingivoperiosteoplasty. Infants with wide unilateral cleft lip and palate can be mesenchymally deficient, and compressing alveolar cleft with molding and gingivoperiosteoplasty would constrict the arch (Figs 10.1 and 10.2).

Isolated clefts of primary palate due to bony fusion of the secondary palate the alveolar segments are more resistant to presurgical molding. Bilateral clefts are difficult to align.

## PRIMARY BONE GRAFTING

Alveolar bone grafting[3] at the time of primary dentition before 2 years of age, primary bone grafting was advocated in mid 20th Century by Schmid and

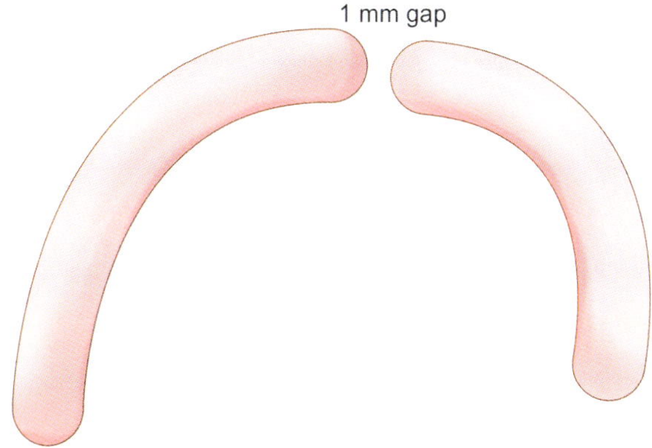

**Fig. 10.1:** Gingivoperiosteoplasty

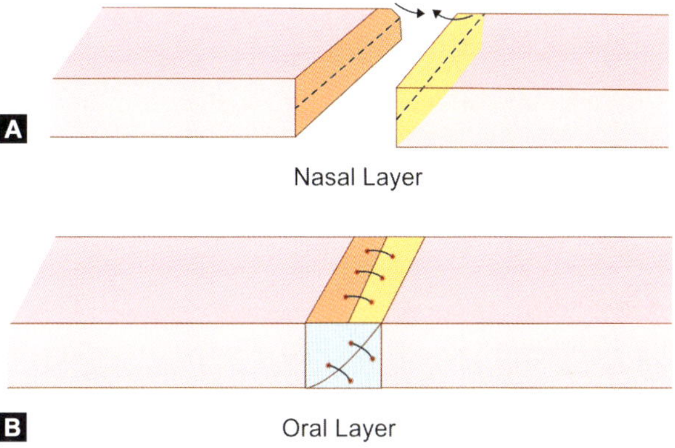

**Fig. 10.2:** Closure of nasal and oral layer of alveolus

others. Long-term follow-up shows iotrogenic impairment of facial growth. Rosenstein and Dado have used primary bone grafting for 20 years. Maxillary appliance is used prior to lip repair to align the alveolar segments. Lip repair was done at the age of 3 months. The appliance is rearranged to prevent posterior collapse of arch. Once approximation is achieved, autogenous split rib graft is used for stabilization and appliance is continued thereafter.

## SECONDARY BONE GRAFTING[4,5]

Secondary bone grafting with autogenous cancellous bone graft at the time of mixed dentition between 6 years and 12 years of age is gold standard treatment. A stable healed graft prior to canine eruption results in superior bone environment. Successful eruption of cuspid through the graft occurred when root formation of the canine adjacent to the cleft was one-fourth to one-half formed at the time of graft placement. Primary teeth adjacent to the cleft should be extracted 3–6 weeks prior to bone grafting. Preoperative arch expansion achieve alignment of maxillary arches. A superiorly based mucoperiosteal flap is raised off the lesser segment of alveolus in subperiosteal flap. Labial mucosa is released up to the superior extent of the alveolar cleft nasolabial fistula. Oronasal fistula is closed. Corticocancellous bone graft is harvested from iliac crest. Cortical strut is used to reconstruct the pyriform rim. Cancellous bone graft is placed in gap over deficient maxillary bone. Oral layer is closed. Expansion of arch should wait for 6–10 weeks. If may take several months or even a year before the canine tooth erupts through the new bone graft.

## LATE SECONDARY BONE GRAFTING

Late secondary bone grafting, after eruption of permanent dentition, 12 years of age does not correct periodontal defects. The goal of grafting is to provide support for prosthetic placement. Corticocancellous graft is fixed with titanium implants.

## BONE MORPHOGENIC PROTEIN

Use of $rhBMP_2$ in treatment of alveolar cleft have shown improved bone healing and reduced donor morbidity and cost compared to those filled with autologus iliac crest bone graft. Ectopic bone formation, bone resorption, hematoma, painful seroma and neck swelling are reported complication.

## REFERENCES


1. Harmada Y, Kondoh T, Noguchi K, et al. Application of limited Cone beam computed tomography to clinical assessment of alveolar bone grafting : A preliminary report. Cleft Palate Craniofac. J. 2005;42:128-37.
2. Iino M, Ishii H, Matsushima R, et al. Comparison of intraoral radiography and computed tomography in evaluation of formation of bone after grafting for repair of residual alveolar defects in patients with cleft lip and palate. Scand J Plast Reconstr Surg Hand Surg. 2005; 39:15-21.
3. Samb G. Effect of alveolar bone grafting on maxillary growth in unilateral cleft lip and palate. Cleft Palate J. 1988;25:288-95.
4. A byholm FE, Berlard O, Semb G. Secondary bone grafting of alveolar clefts. A surgical/orthodontic treatment enabling a nonprosthodontic rehabilitation in cleft lip and palate patients. Scand J Plast Reconstr Surg. 1981;15:127-40.
5. Long Jr RE, Spanglar BE, Yow M. Cleft width and secondary alveolar bone graft success. Cleft Palate Craniofac J. 1995;32:420-27.

# CHAPTER 11

# Secondary Deformities of the Cleft Lip, Nose and Palate

The secondary deformities of the cleft lip, nose and palate are due to multiple factors.[1] They are influenced by the type and severity of the cleft, preoperative analysis, primary surgery timing and technique, postoperative care and orthodontic treatment. Correction of clefts leads to restriction of growth of midface as once thought, now research suggests hypoplasia may be secondary to an intrinsic growth deficit. Physical growth, fourth dimension in cleft lip and palate surgery is difficult to predict.

## CLEFT LIP

Scarring of lip may be improved with moisturization cream and silicone based gel. Local steroid injection may be helpful. Scar revision surgeries and Z-plasty may be helpful for better cosmetic outcome.

Vermilion deformities like thin or thick lip segments, vermilion notching, vermilion mismatches, border malalignment or whistle deformity are common. Improper muscle approximation during primary repair or subsequent dehiscence presents bulge in the lateral aspect of repair. Buccal sulcus deformity due to scar contracture or from true paucity of tissue needs correction.[2] Short lip, long lip, tight lip, wide lip and short lateral lip segments are corrected at the ages of 5–6 years (Figs 11.1 to 11.11).

## CLEFT PALATE FISTULA

Palatal fistulas are significant complications after cleft palate surgery.[3-7] Cleft palate fistula may have no symptoms, increased nasal air emission, hypernasal speech and nasal regurgitation of fluid or food. Fistulas are classified by Pittsburgh fistula classification system.

*Types of fistula*
1. Uvula
2. Soft palate
3. Soft-hard palate junction

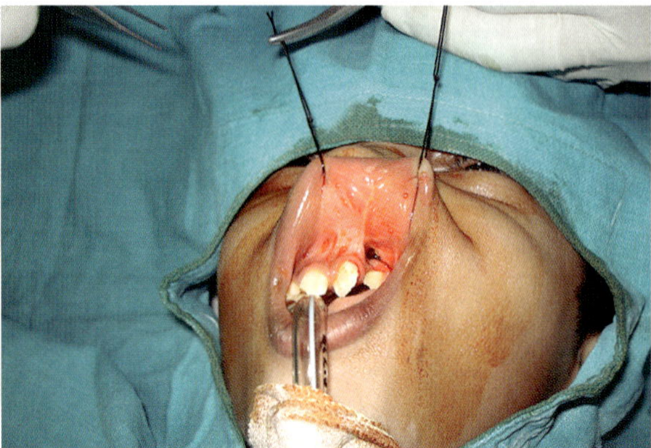

**Fig. 11.1:** Left complete cleft lip with palate (operated)—nasolabial fistula

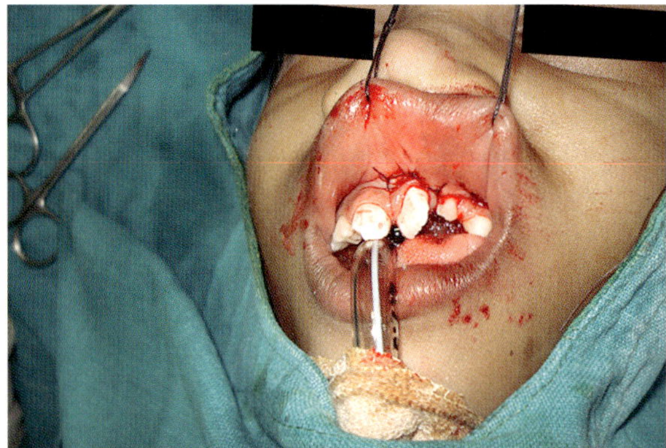

**Fig. 11.2:** Nasolabial fistula was closed in two layers

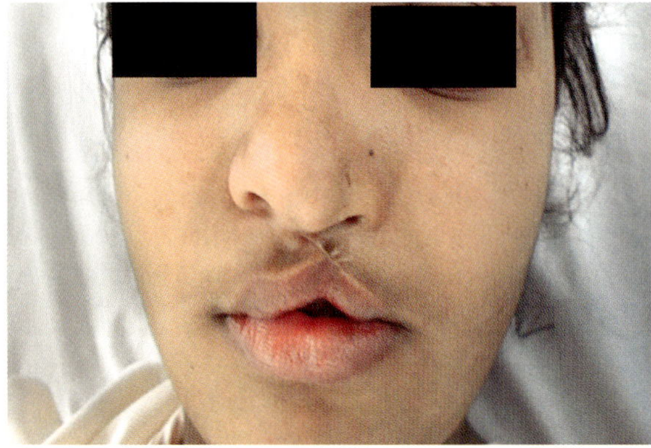

**Fig. 11.3:** Left complete cleft lip (operated) having notching of vermilion

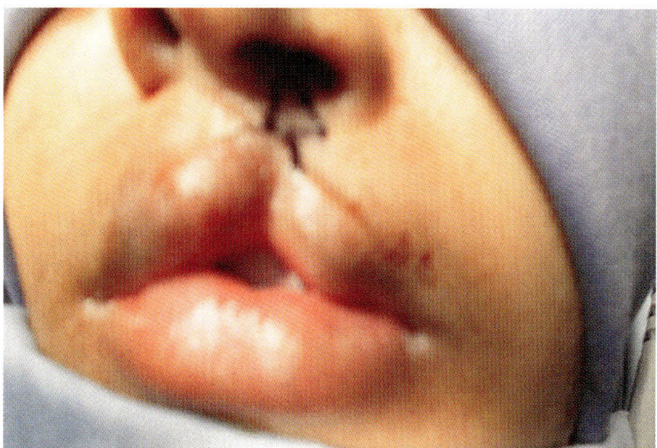

**Fig. 11.4:** Triangular flap planned

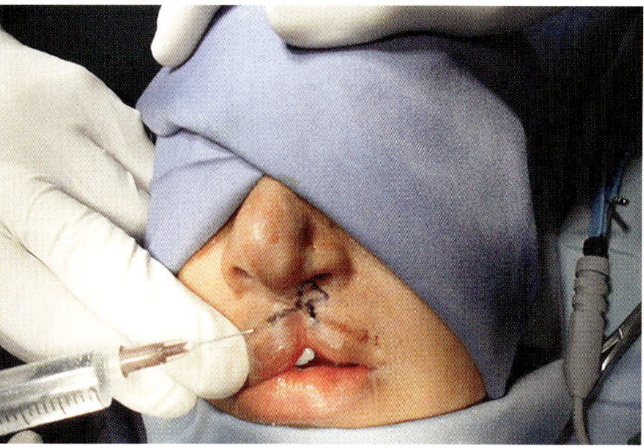

**Fig. 11.5:** Xylocaine with adrenaline was injected locally

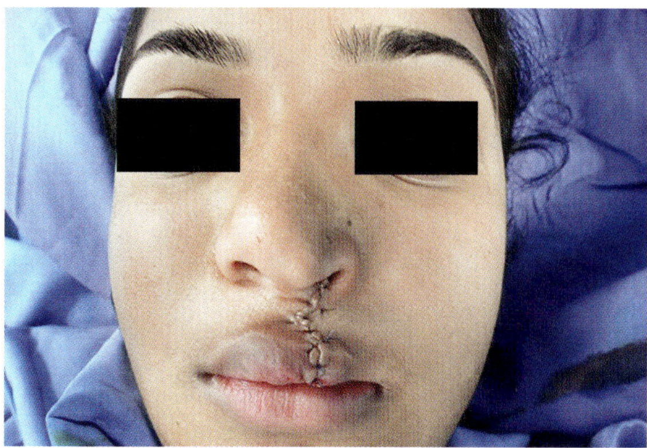

**Fig. 11.6:** Repair completed

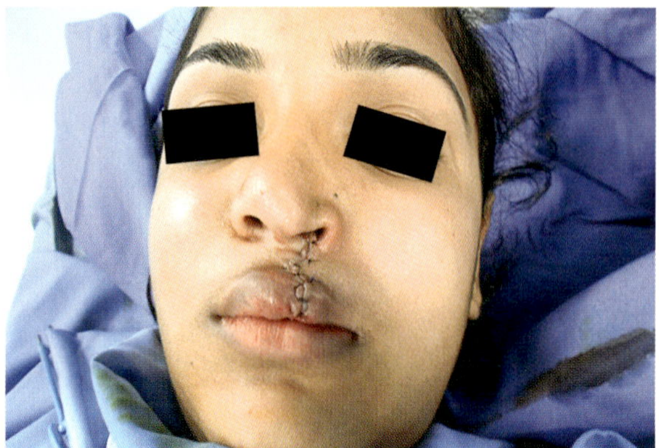

**Fig. 11.7:** Triangular flap was used to increase height of lip

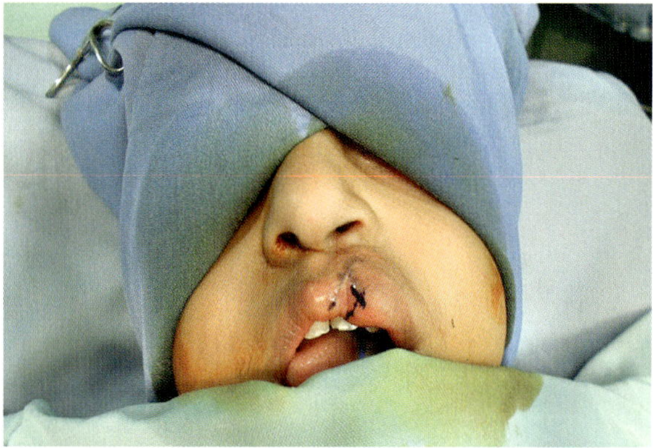

**Fig. 11.8:** Vermilion notching

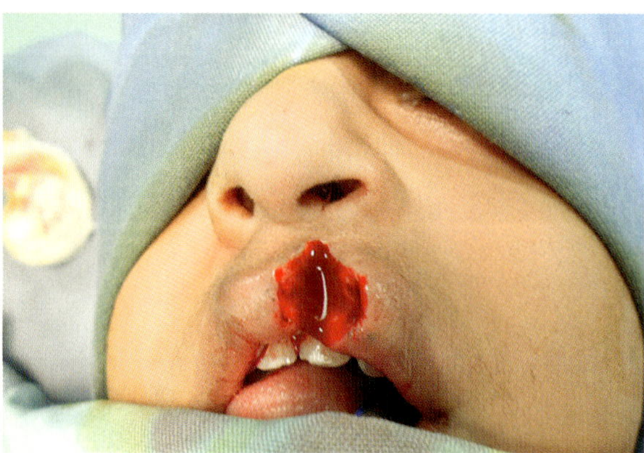

**Fig. 11.9:** V-excision done

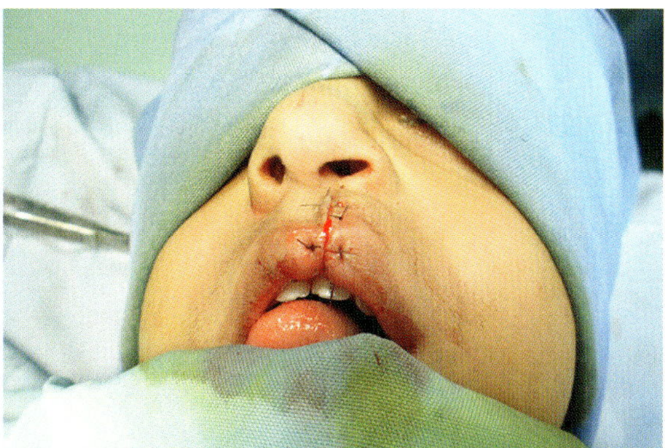

**Fig. 11.10:** 4-0 vicryl used for muscle and mucosa closure and 6-0 nylon for skin closure

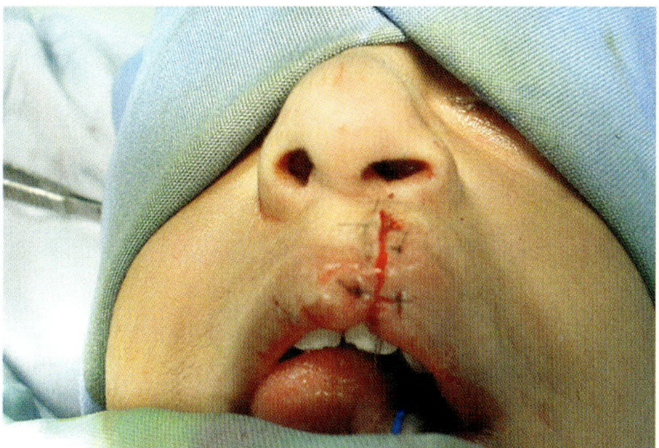

**Fig. 11.11:** Height of lip and vermilion border alignment was achieved

4. Hard palate
5. Incisive foramen
6. Lingual alveolar
7. Labial alveolar.

   Fistulas are closed with local flap,[8] buccal mucosal flap,[9] tongue flap,[10] posterior pharyngeal flap, or free flap (Figs 11.12 to 11.16).[11,12]

## CLEFT NOSE[13,14]

Secondary rhinoplasty is performed at the age of 14–16 years in cleft patients (Figs 11.17 to 11.31).

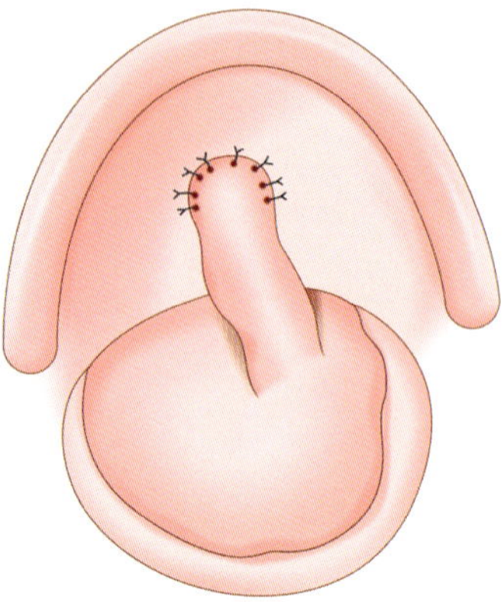

**Fig. 11.12:** Tongue flap for palatal fistula closure

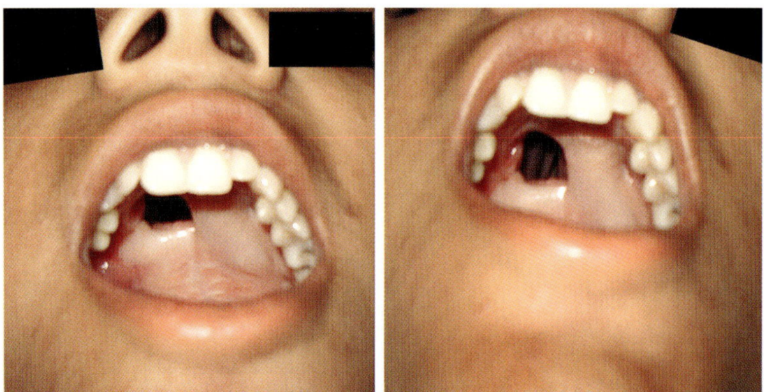

**Fig. 11.13:** Cleft palate large fistula

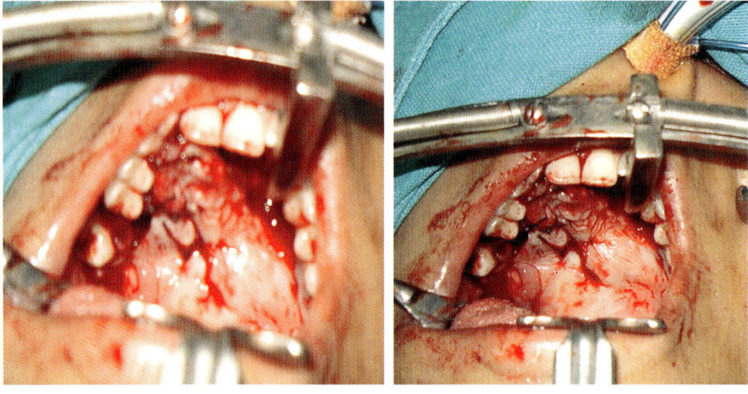

**Fig. 11.14:** Fistula repaired with two long flaps

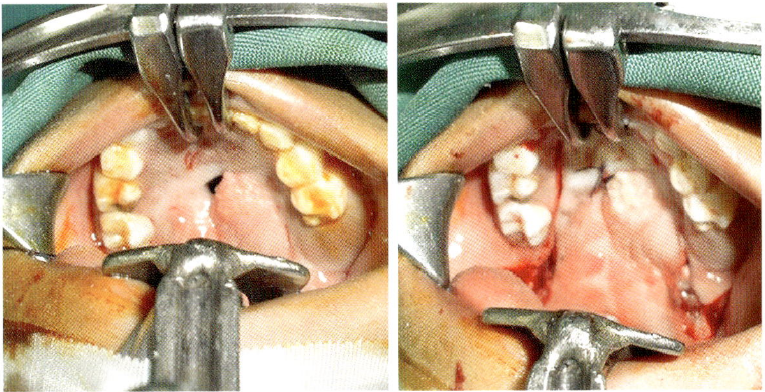

**Fig. 11.15:** Palatal fistula repaired with von Langenbeck flap

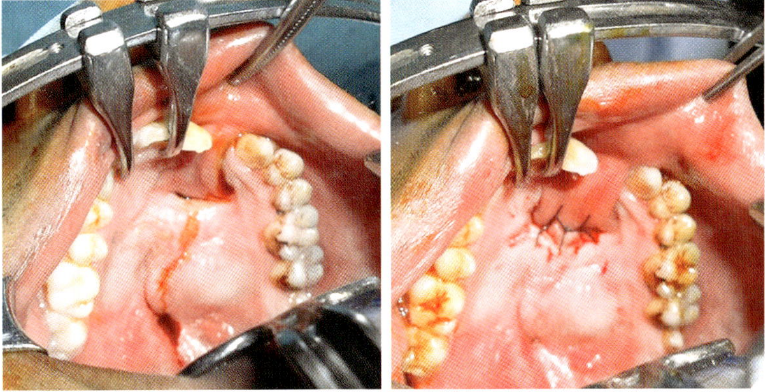

**Fig. 11.16:** Anterior cleft palate fistula repaired with labial advancement flap

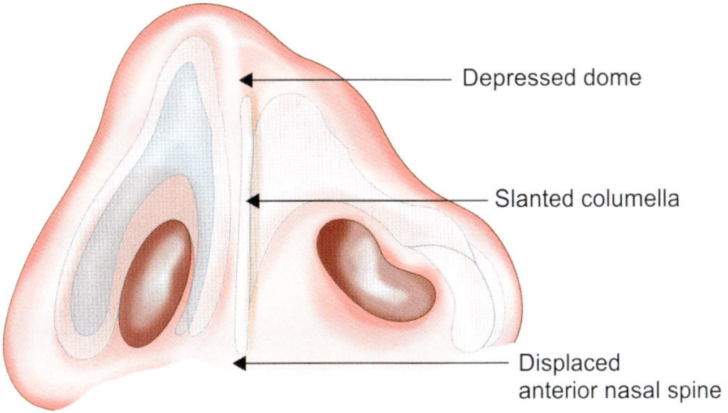



**Fig. 11.17:** Anatomy of unilateral cleft lip nose

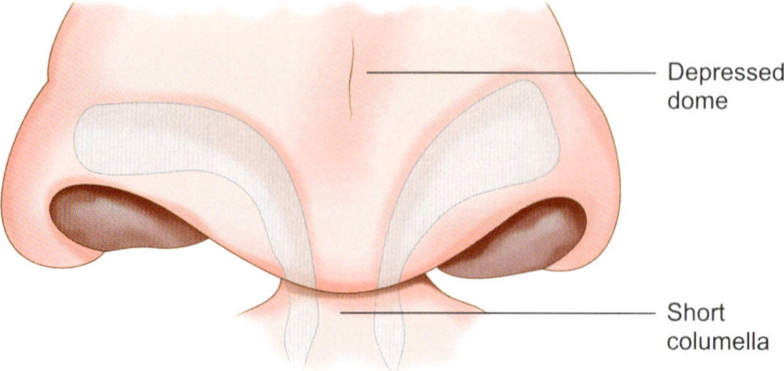



**Fig. 11.18:** Anatomy of bilateral cleft lip nose[15]

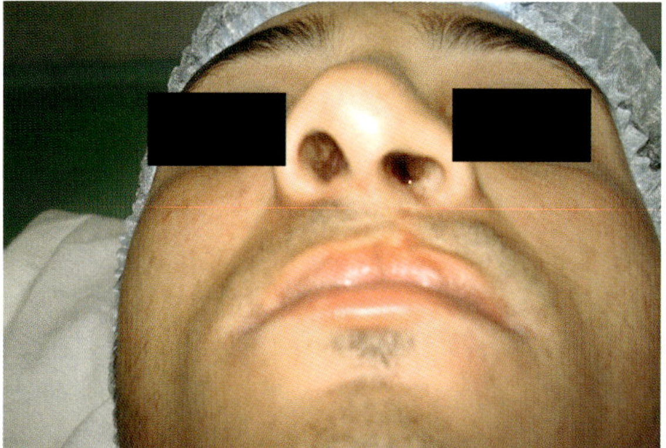

**Fig. 11.19:** Left unilateral cleft lip (operated) with nasal deformities

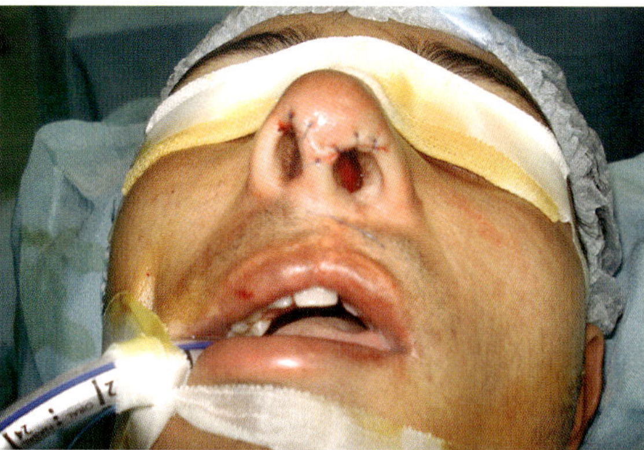

**Fig. 11.20:** Flying bird rim incision taken, flap is elevated, medial crura of alar cartilage are sutured together with 6-0 prolene. If there is fat between two medial crura, fat is existed first before suturing crura together. If depression still persists over tip conchal cartilage graft is placed over tip

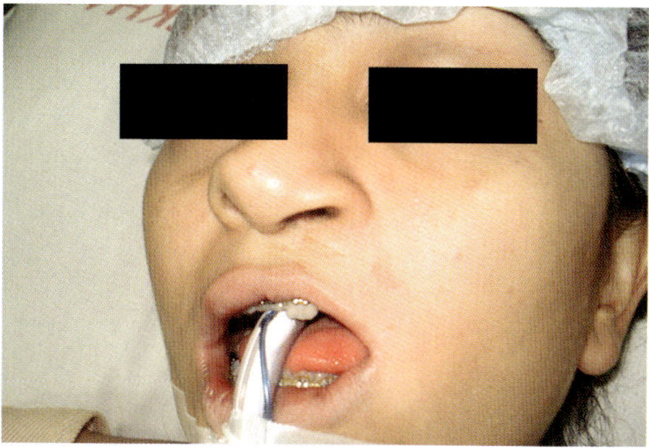

**Fig. 11.21:** A case of left unilateral cleft lip with palate (operated) having nasal deformities

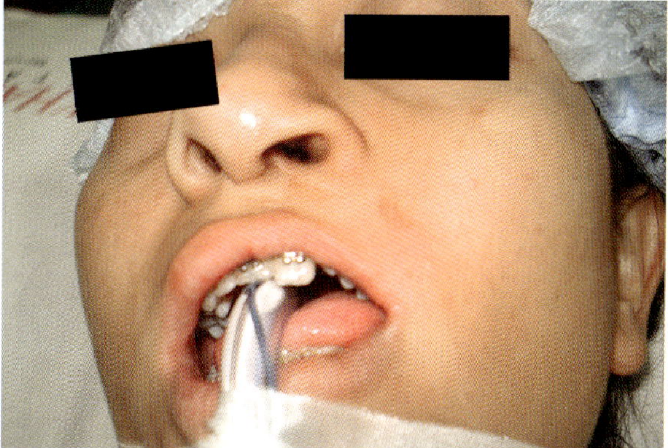

**Fig. 11.22:** Worm's view of nasal deformity of left unilateral cleft lip

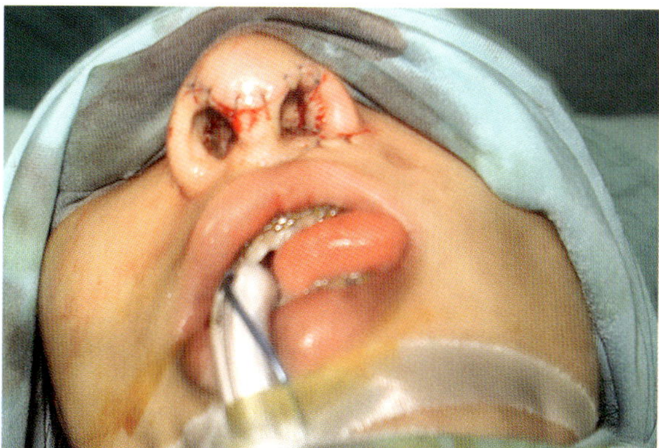

**Fig. 11.23:** Postoperative worm's view

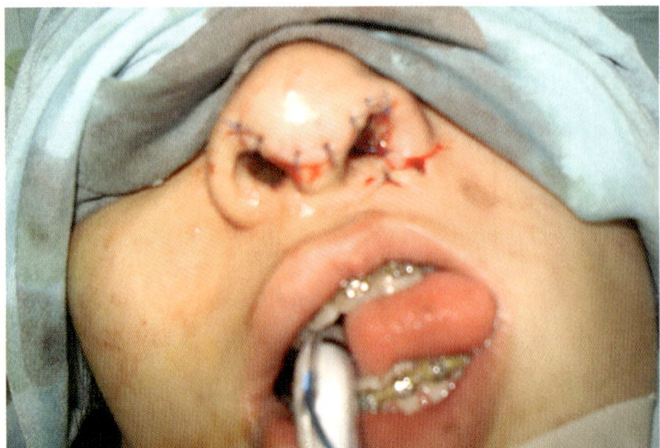

**Fig. 11.24:** Left alae was shifted medially with Y–V plasty

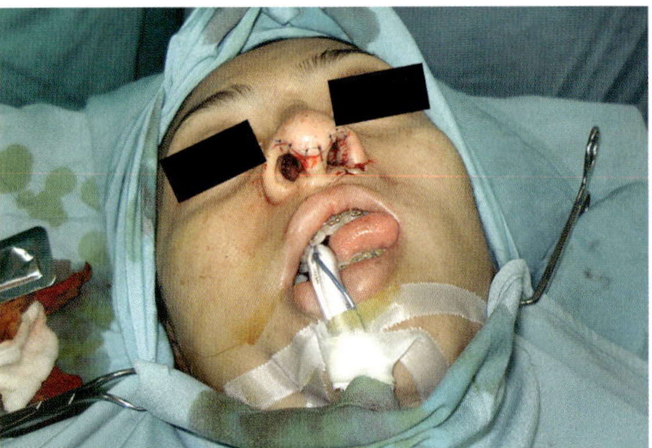

**Fig. 11.25:** Left alar base was transposed medially

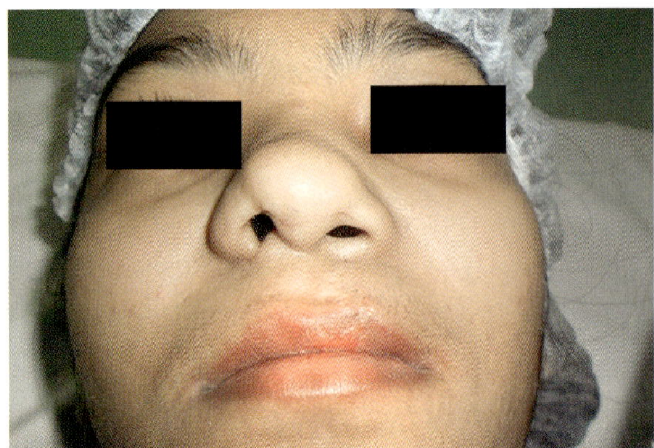

**Fig. 11.26:** A patient with depressed left alar region due to maxillary hypoplasia in left unilateral cleft lip with palate

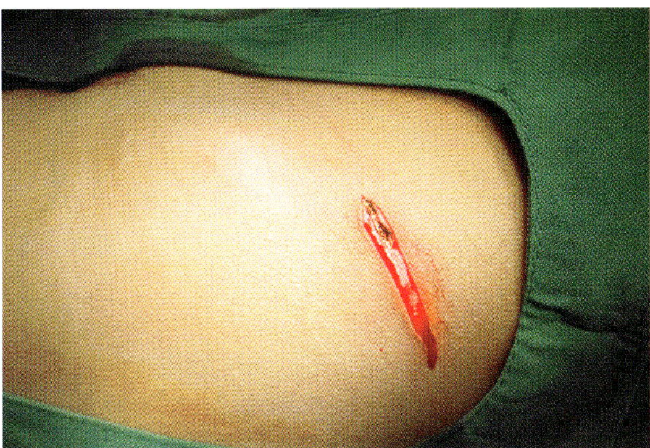

**Fig. 11.27:** Iliac crest bone graft harvested

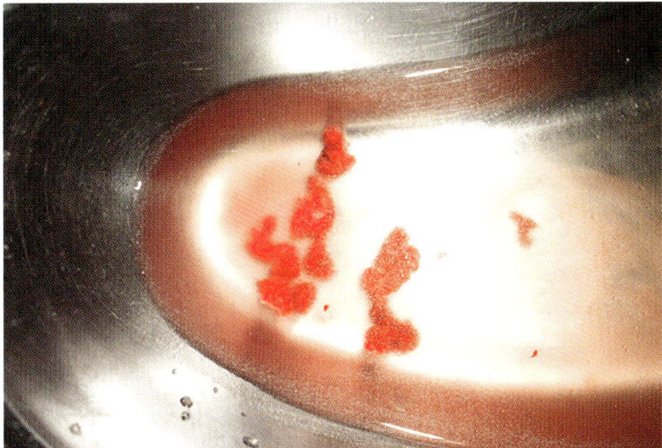

**Fig. 11.28:** Corticocancellous graft is harvested from right iliac crest

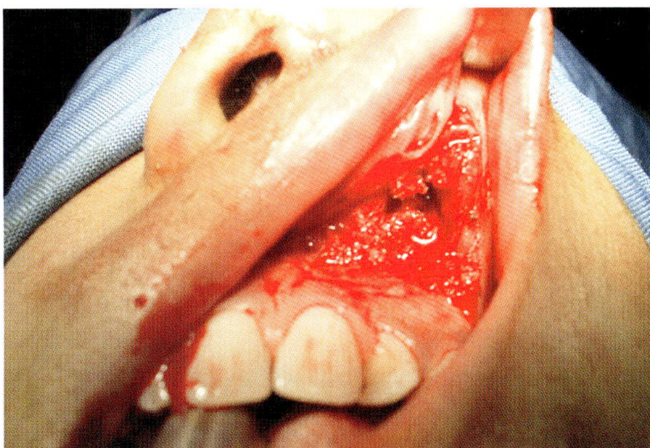

**Fig. 11.29:** Through buccal sulcus incision corticocancellous grafts is placed in front of maxilla to elevate alar region

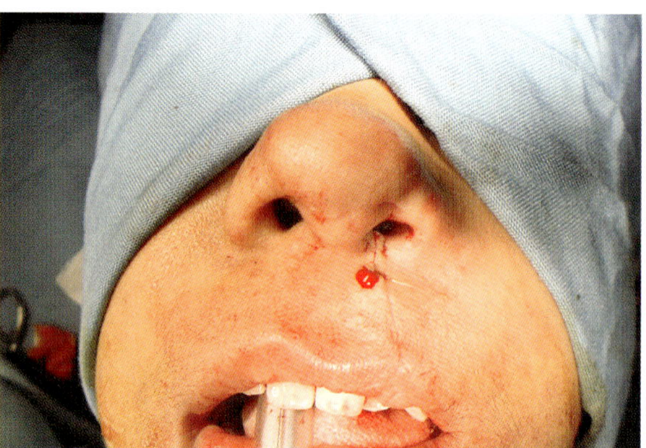

**Fig. 11.30:** Laterally displaced left alar region was brought medially

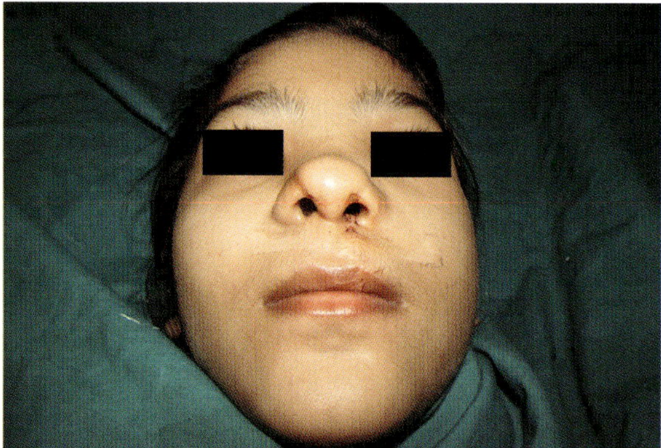

**Fig. 11.31:** Wounds heal well and patient had good cosmetic output

## REFERENCES


1. Brand S, Blechschmidt A, Muller A, et al. Psychosocial functioning and sleep patterns in children and adolescents with cleft lip and palate compared with healthy controls. Cleft Palate Craniofac J. 2009;46:124-35.
2. Erol OO, Agaoglu G. Reconstruction of the superior labial sulcus in secondary bilateral cleft lip deformities. An invented U-shaped flap. Plast Reconstr Surg. 2001;108:1871-3.
3. Ashtiani AK, Emami SA, Rasti M. Closure of complicated palatal fistula with facial artery musculomucous flap. Plast Reconstr Surg. 2005;116:381-6.
4. Bozola AR, Gasques JA, Carriquiry CE, et al. The buccinator musculomucosal flap: anatomic study and clinical application. Plast Reconstr Surg. 1989;84:250-7.
5. Noor SFM, Musa S. Assessment of patients level of satisfaction with cleft treatment using the cleft evaluation profile. Cleft Palate Cranioface. 2007;44:292-303.
6. Cohen SR, Kalinowski J, LaRossa D, et al. Cleft palate fistula : a multivariate statistical analysis of prevalence, etiology and surgical management. Plast Reconstr Surg. 1991;87:1041-7.

7. Van Der Wal KGH, Mulda JW. The temporal muscle flap for closure of large palatal defects in CLP patients. Int J Oral Maxillofac Surg. 1992;21:3-5.
8. Denny AD, Amm CA. Surgical technique for the correction of postpalatoplasty fistulae of the hard palate. Plast Reconstr Surg. 2005;115:383-7.
9. Robertson AGN, Mckeown DJ, Bello-Rojas G, et al. Use of buccal myomucosal flap in secondary cleft palate repair. Plast Reconstr Surg. 1989;84:250-7.
10. Assuncao AGA. The design of tongue flaps for the closure of palatal fistulas. Plats Reconstr Surg. 1993;91:806-10.
11. Chen H, Ganos DL, Coessens BC, et al. Free forearm flap for closure of difficult oronasal fistulas in cleft palate patients. Plast Reconstr Surg. 1992;90:757-62.
12. Hallock GG. Repair of an untreated cleft palate in an adult using a prefabricated redial forearm flap. Ann Plast Surg. 1997;38:69-73.
13. Gruber RP, Freedman GD. Suture algorithm for the broad or bulbous nasal tip. Plast Reconstr Surg. 2002;110:1752-64.
14. Warrer DW, Drake AF. Cleft nose; form and function clin. Plast Surg. 1993;20:769-79.
15. Van der Meulen JC. Columellar elongation in bilateral cleft lip repair. Early results. Plast Reconstr Surg.1992;89:1060-7.

# CHAPTER 12

# Nasal Conformer and Nasoalveolar Molding

## INTRODUCTION

Nasal conformer[1-3] is used for presurgical molding for patients having incomplete cleft lip. It increases height of columella. Nasal conformer is used for postoperative maintenance of nasal configuration. Height of silicone nasal conformer can be increased by adding layer of soft resin or silicone sheets on the dome (Figs 12.1 to 12.5).

**Presurgical nasoalveolar molding:** The presurgical nasoalveolar molding[4,5] is to restore a more normal nasal shape and a balanced skeletal base. Patients are advised to sleep either prone or side lying position to increase pressure on cheek. It is important to start using nasoalveolar molding technique[6,7] earlier preferably within first two weeks of birth (Figs 12.6 to 12.9).

## GRAYSON'S TECHNIQUE[8,9]

The protruding premaxilla is molded first into proper position with passive type of orthopedic appliances and tapping of the lip in bilateral cleft lip and palate and alveolar approximation in unilateral cleft lip with palate. A nasal

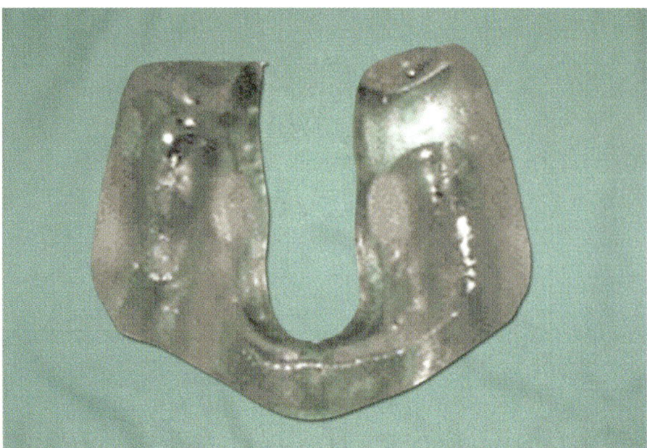

**Fig. 12.1:** Nasal Conformer – Silicone

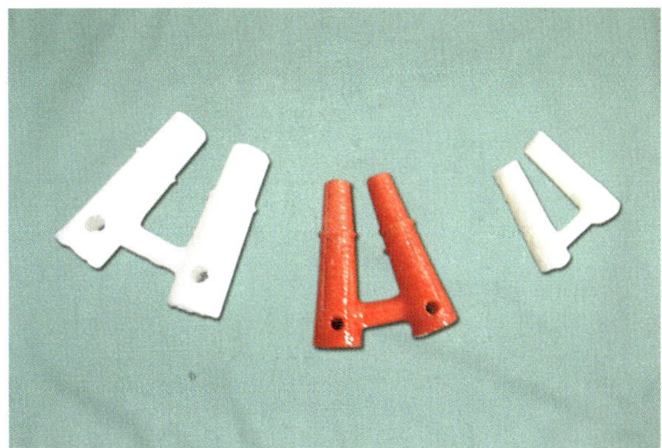

**Fig. 12.2:** Nasal conformer

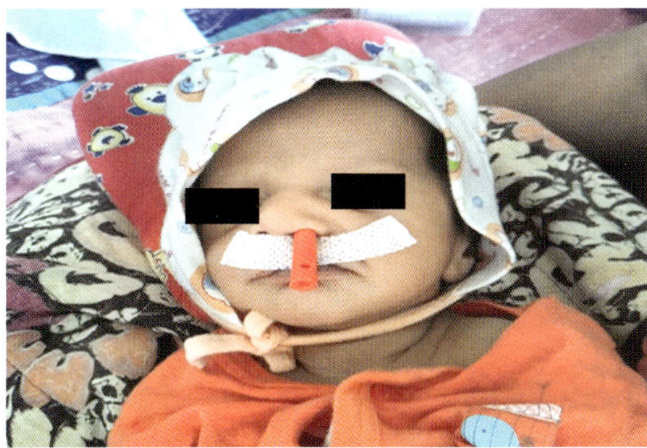

**Fig. 12.3:** Nasal conformer for preoperative nasal molding

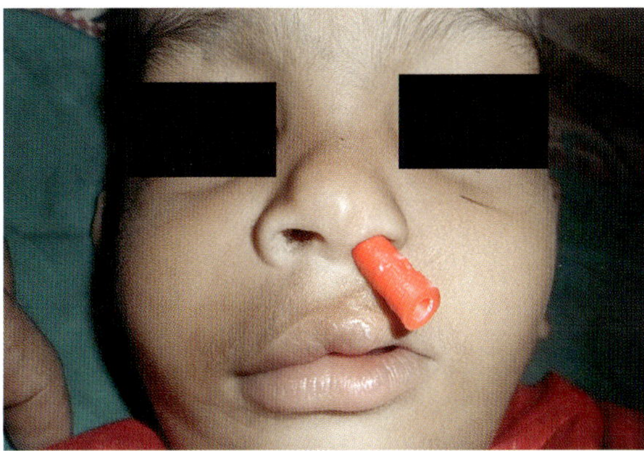

**Fig. 12.4:**

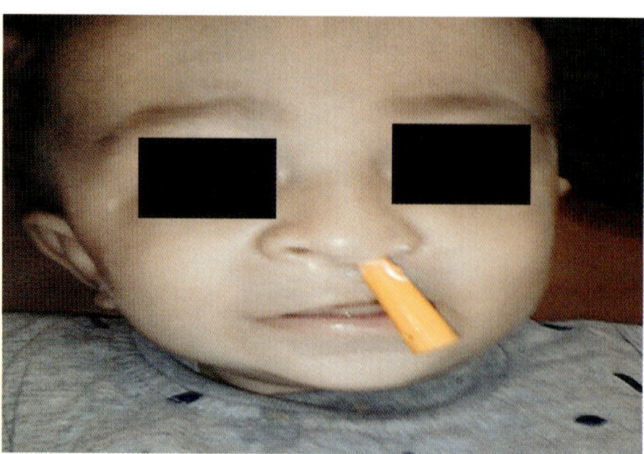

**Figs 12.4 and 12.5:** Nasal conformer for postoperative nasal molding

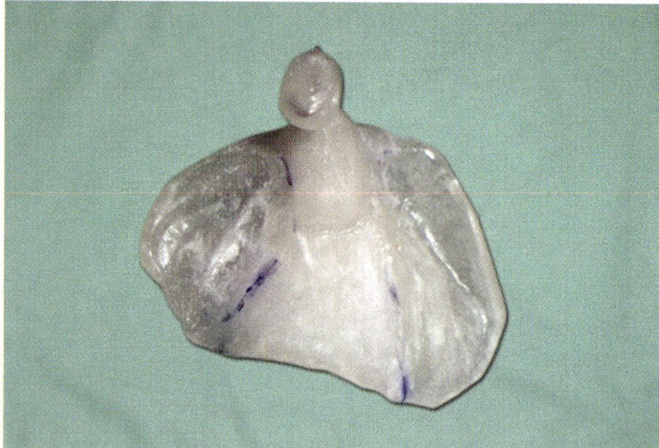

**Fig. 12.6:**

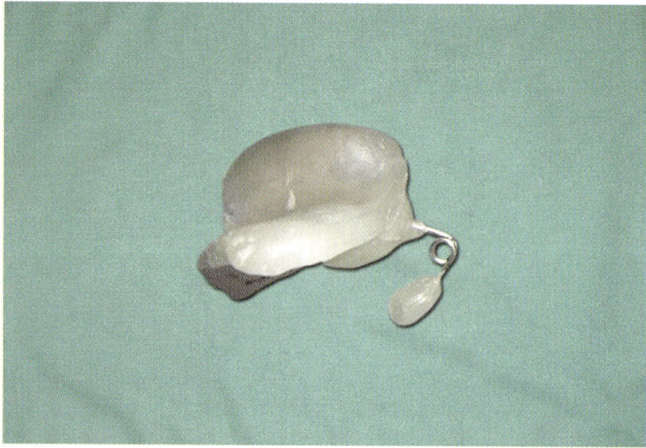

**Figs 12.6 and 12.7:** Nasoalveolar molding

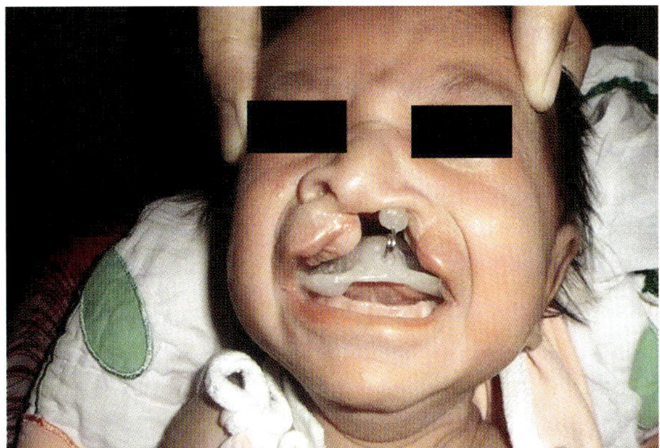

**Fig. 12.8:** Nasoalveolar molding in place

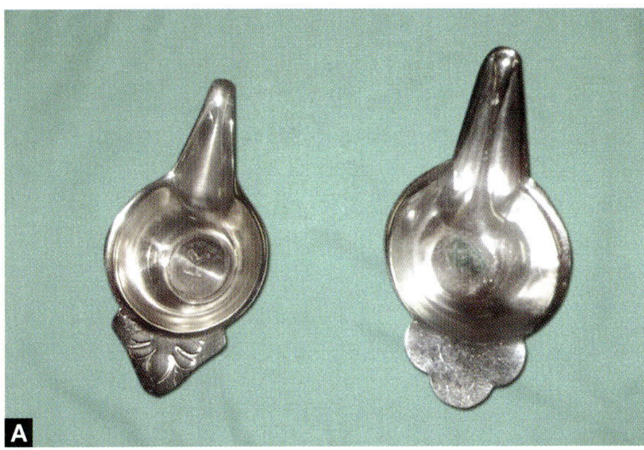

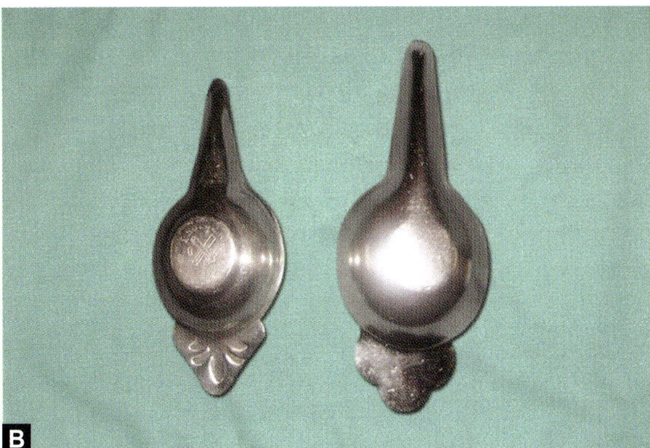

**Figs 12.9:** Vessel for feeding cleft cases

molding device is added to orthopedic appliances to increase the columellar length, reshape alar dome. This two-stage procedure avoid overstretching of nasal cartilage.

## FIGUERA'S TECHNIQUE

Alveolar molding and nasal molding are performed simultaneously with an acrylic plate and rigid acrylic nasal extension. A soft resin ball attached to acrylic plate across the prolabium maintains nasolabial angle. Rubber bands help gentle retraction of premaxilla backwards.

## LIOU'S TECHNIQUE[10,11]

The nasoalveolar molding device is composed of a dental plate, nasal component for nasal molding and micropore taps for premaxillary retraction. Dental plates are kept on lateral maxillary segments with dental adhesive. Nasal components are made up of stainless steel wire and soft resin molding bulb that fits underneath the nasal cartilage. It increases columellar height and supports nasal tip and cartilages.

## REFERENCES


1. Nakajima T, Yoshimura Y, Sakakibara A. Augmentation of the nostril splint for retaining the corrected contour of the cleft lip nose. Plast Reconstr Surg. 1990;85:182-6.
2. Osada M, Hashimoto K, Akiyama T. Application of intra and extranasal silicone prosthesis after the operation of nasal deformities. J Plast Reconstr Surg. 1969;11:191.
3. Yeow VK, Chen PK, Chen YR, et al. The use of nasal splints in the primary management of unilateral cleft nasal deformity. Plast Reconstr Surg. 1999;103(5): 1347-54.
4. Barillas I, Dec W, Warren SM, et al. Nasoalveolar molding improves long-term nasal symmetry in complete unilateral cleft lip-cleft palate patients. Plast Reconstr Surg. 2009;123(3):1002-6.
5. Pai BC, Ko EW, Huang CS, et al. Symmetry of the nose after presurgical nasoalveolar molding in infants with unilateral cleft lip and palate: a preliminary study. Cleft Palate Craniofac J. 2005;42(6):658-63.
6. Singh GD, Levy-Bercowski D, Santiago PE. Three-dimensional nasal changes following nasoalveolar molding in patients with unilateral cleft lip and palate: geometric morphometrics. Cleft Palate Craniofac J. 2005;42(4):403-9.
7. Winter JC, Hurwitz DJ. Presurgical orthopaedics in the surgical management of unilateral cleft lip and palate. Plast Reconstr Surg. 1995;95:755-64.
8. Grayson BH, Santiago PE, Brecht LE, et al. Presurgical nasoalveolar molding in infants with cleft lip and palate. Cleft Palate Craniofac. 1999;36:486-98.
9. Grayson BH, Garfinkle JS. Nasoalveolar molding and columellar elongation in preparation for primary repair of unilateral cleft lip and bilateral cleft lip and palate. In: Losee JE, (Ed). Comprehensive cleft care. New York, McGraw-Hill. 2009:701-20.
10. Liou EJ, Subramanian M, Chen PK, et al. The progressive changes of nasal symmetry and growth after nasoalveolar molding: a three-year follow-up study. Plast Reconstr Surg. 2004;114(4):858-64.
11. Liou EJ, Subramanian M, Chen PK. Progressive changes of columella length and nasal growth after nasoalveolar molding in bilateral cleft patients: a 3-years follow-up study. Plast Reconstr Surg. 2007;119:642-8.

# CHAPTER 13

# Orthodontic Treatment and Orthognathic Surgery for Cleft Patients

## PRIMARY DENTITION

Orthodontic treatment[1-3] is advised to correct posterior crossbites and anterior crossbites of mild-to-moderate degree. Posterior crossbites are of skeletal and dental origin. Post-cleft palate surgery there is collapse of maxillary segments, particularly in canine region. Primary canine erupts medially to the lower one. Liou and Tsai advocated spring system with highly flexible wires to apply constant pressure to the maxilla. Screw type expander is regularly activated and it is turned backwards once it reaches its limit. This maneuver results in activation of the circum maxillary suture complex and maxillary protraction is gained.

## TRANSITIONAL DENTITION

The dentition around cleft present severe malposition limiting surgical access to the alveolar site. The dentition adjacent to the cleft needs the reposition for secondary alveolar bone grafting. Orthodontic treatment should be initiated after the near complete the root development of the incisors on which orthodontic brackets will be placed. The development of cleft lateral incisor is delayed. Bonded edgewise appliances correct first stage. New self-ligating brackets and highly flexible orthodontic arch wires helps slow and highly efficient tooth movement. Occasionally, maxilla expander is used for expansion of arch.

Secondary alveolar bone grafting is done after maxillary segments and dentition are placed in their ideal positions. Orthodontic treatment can be restarted after 8–12 weeks of bone grafting. Orthodontic appliances are removed after achieving appropriate maxillary arch and dental relations. Removable prosthetic appliances used for absent teeth to improve esthetics.

## PERMANENT DENTITION

Definitive orthodontic treatment[4-6] is given at time of permanent dentition phase. Dental extraction is carried out in case of severe crowding. Congenitally, missing teeth or severely abnormal teeth that may need to be extracted requiring either replacement with a prosthesis or with orthodontic space closure particularly in cleft region. Self-ligating appliances and flexible wires helps achieve class 1 cuspid and molar relationships with ideal overjet and overbite. Bone anchoring screws permits anteroposterior and vertical control of a single tooth or group of the teeth.

Patients with cleft developed class 3 malocclusion due to maxillary retrusion. Orthognathic surgery is performed after the complete facial growth. Class 2 occlusion anterior crossbite or posterior crossbite can also occur. Treatment should favor expansive anterior and inferior repositioning to achieve class 1 occlusion.

Team consists of plastic surgeons, otorhinolaryngologist, dentist and speech therapist evaluate patients. Patients may develop hypernasality after post-maxillary advancement. Cephalometric and dental evaluation, model surgery and 3D CT modeling improves accuracy in treatment.

## LEFORT 1 OSTEOTOMY[7–12]

The vertical position of maxilla is distance between the medial canthus and orthodontic archwires. Under general anesthesia, with local xylocaine with adrenaline injection incision is kept 5 mm above the mucogingival junction from first molar to first molar. With reciprocating saw transverse osteotomy is performed from the piriform aperture laterally to just posterior to the last maxillary molar and drops through the maxillary tuberosity.[13,14] The cut should be 5 mm above the tooth apices. Descending palatine artery is clipped prophylactically, the maxilla is downfractured. Mandibulomaxillary fixation[2,15] is applied with 26 gauge wires. Four 2 mm plates, L-shaped are used to secure maxilla. Mucosa is sutured with 4-0 vicryl (Figs 13.1 and 13.2).

Surgically assisted rapid palatal expansion procedure offers better maxillary expansion (Fig. 13.3).

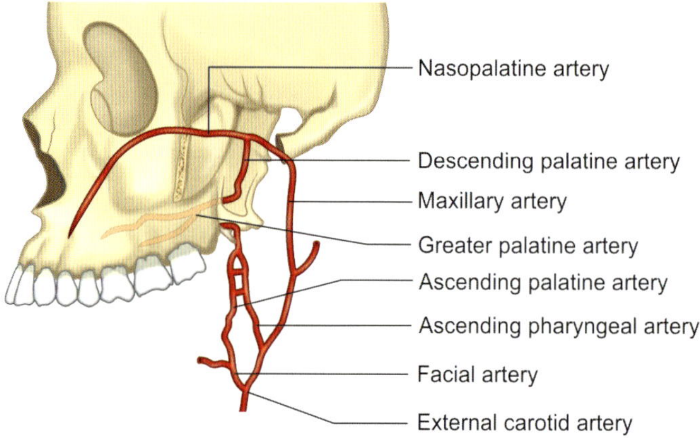


**Fig. 13.1:** Vascular anatomy of maxillae for Lefort 1 osteotomy

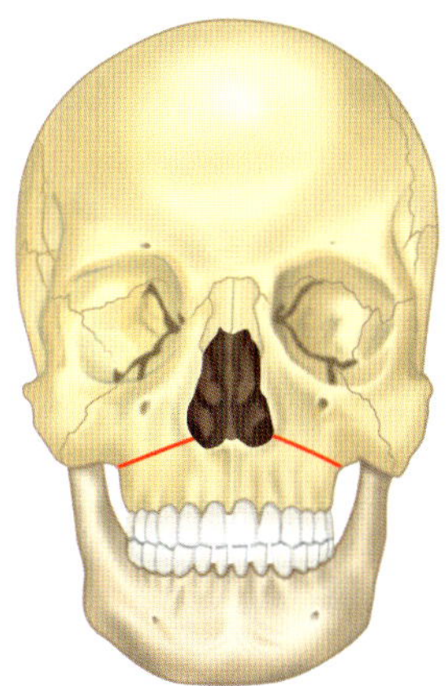

**Fig. 13.2:** Lefort 1 osteotomy

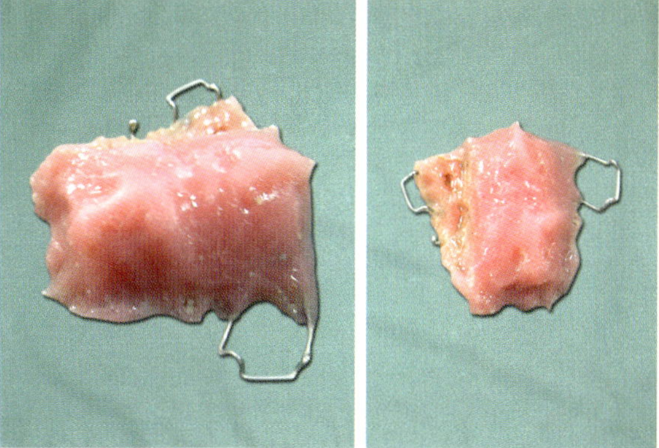

**Fig. 13.3:** Palatal expansion plate

## REFERENCES


1. Aduss H, Figueroa AA. Stages of orthodontic treatment in complete unilateral cleft lip and palate. In: Bardach J, Morris HL, (Eds). Multidisciplinary management of cleft lip and palate. Philadelphia: WB Saunders. 1990:607-15.
2. Losse J, Kirsehner RE, (Eds). Comprehensive cleft care. New York: McGraw-Hill. 2009:721-47.
3. Mercado A, Vig KWL. Orthodontic principles in the management of orthofacial clefts. In: Losee J, Kirschner RE, (Eds). Comprehensive cleft care. New York: McGraw-Hill. 2009:721-47.
4. Fergueroa A, Aduss H. Orthodontic management for patients with cleft lip and palate. In: Cohen M, (Ed). Mastery of plastic and reconstructive surgery. Boston: Little, Brown. 1994;648-68.
5. Figueroa AA, Polley JW, Cohen M. Orthodontic management of cleft lip and palate patient. CL: Plast Surg. 1993;20:733-53.

6. Harada K, Baba Y, Ohyama K, et al. Soft tissue profile changes of the midface in patients with cleft lip and palate following maxillary distraction osteogenesis: a preliminary study. Oral Surg Oral Med Oral Pathol Oral Radio Endod. 2002;94;673-7.

7. DeLuke DM, Marchanda A, Robles EC, et al. Facial growth and need for orthognathic surgery after cleft palate repair: Literature review and report of 28 cases. J Oral Maxillofac Surg. 1997;55:694-7;discussion 697-8.

8. Good PM, Mulliken JB, Padwa BL. Frequency of Le Fort 1 Osteotomy after repaired cleft lip/palate or cleft palate. Cleft-Palate Craniofac J. 2007;44:396-401.

9. Ko EW, Figueroa AA, Guyette TW, et al. Velopharyngeal changes after maxillary advancement in cleft patients with distraction osteogenesis using a rigid external distraction device: a 1-year cephalometric follow-up. J Craniofac Surg. 1999;10(4):312-20;discussion 321-2.

10. Obwegeser H. Surgery of the maxilla for the correction of prognathism. SSO Schweiz Monatsschr Zahnheilkd. 1965;75:365-74.

11. Posnick JC, Dagys AP. Skeletal stability and relapse patterns after Lefort 1 maxillary osteotomy fixed with miniplates: The unilateral cleft lip and palate deformity. Plast Reconstr Surg. 1994;94:924-32.

12. Tompach PC, Wheeler JJ, Fridrich KL. Orthodontic considerations in orthognathic surgery. Int J Adult Orthodon Orthognath Surg. 1995;10(2):97-107.

13. Hirano A, Suzuki H. Factors related to relapse after Lefort 1 maxillary advancement osteotomy in patient with cleft lip and palate. Cleft Palate Craniofac J. 2001;38: 1-10.

14. Polly JW, Figueroa AA. Rigid external distraction: Its application in cleft maxillary deformities. Plast Reconstr Surg. 1998;102:1360-72.

15. Lambrecht J. 3D modelling technology in oral and maxillofacial surgery. Chicago: Quintessence, 1995.

# CHAPTER 14

# Rare Craniofacial Cleft

Tessier classified rare craniofacial cleft[1-5] according to numbering system to identify the consistent anatomic pathways of soft tissue and skeletal clefts (Fig. 14.1).

## NUMBER 0[6-8]

The midline soft tissue anomaly may range from mild broadening of philtrum to a true median cleft lip. Median facial clefting produces a characteristic hypertelorism. There is sometimes anterior open bite. The extension of this cleft into cranium constitutes a number 14 cleft (Figs 14.2 and 14.3).

## NUMBER 1

Above the cleft lip, the clefting of alar dome is associated with deviation to the opposite side of the shortened and broadened columella and nasal tip. A cranial extension characterized by a tongue like projection of the frontal hair line delineates the number 13 cleft.

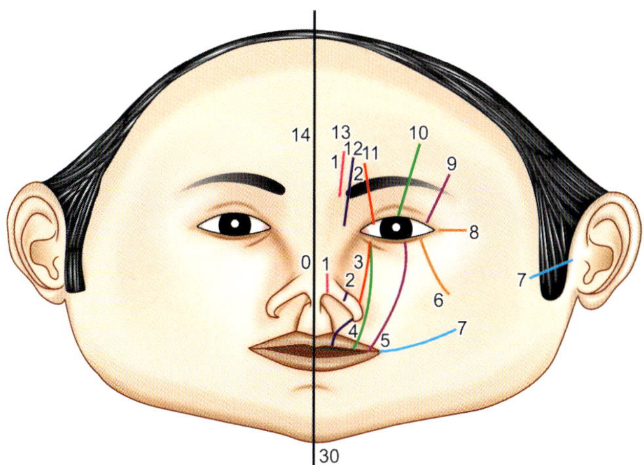


**Fig. 14.1:** Tessier classification of rare craniofacial cleft

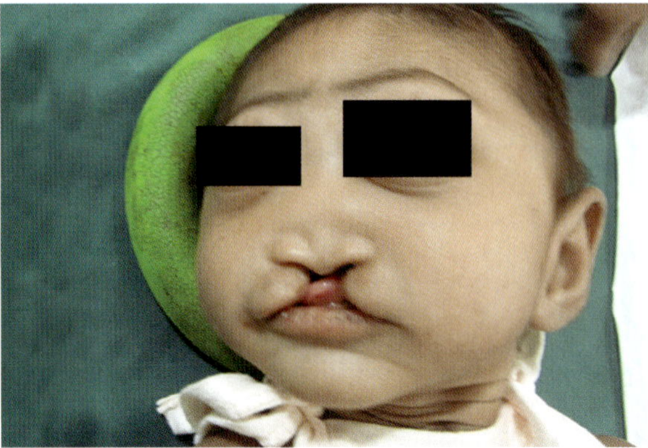

**Fig. 14.2:** Number 0 cleft median craniofacial hypoplasia

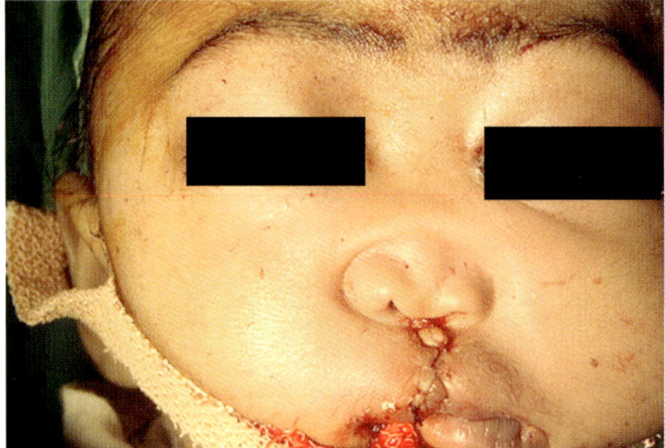

**Fig. 14.3:** Repaired with two small triangular flaps

## NUMBER 2

Above the cleft of the lip and palate, there is broad cleft of the nostril that is medial to the intact but laterally displaced tail of the alar cartilage. There is mild asymmetry of anterior cranial fossa.

## NUMBER 3

There is hypoplasia of the soft tissue margins of the cleft in vertical dimension. This produces soft tissue deficiency between the alar base and the cleft of the medial aspect of the lower eyelid (Figs 14.4 and 14.5).

## NUMBER 4

There is severe vertical soft tissue deficiency with the medial margins of the cleft lip extending directly into the medially placed cleft of the lower eyelid.

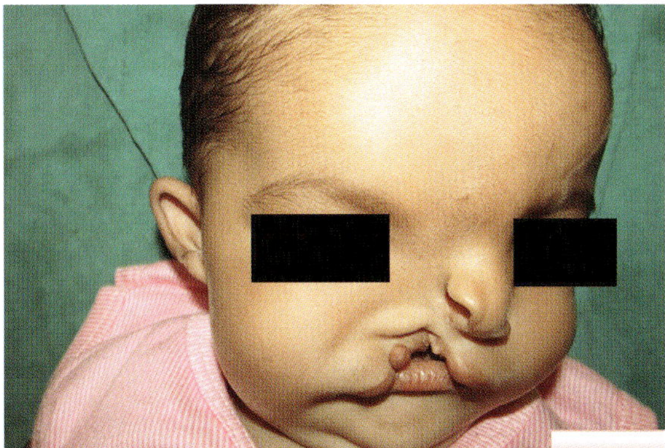

**Fig. 14.4:** Number 3 cleft tessier oronaso-ocular cleft

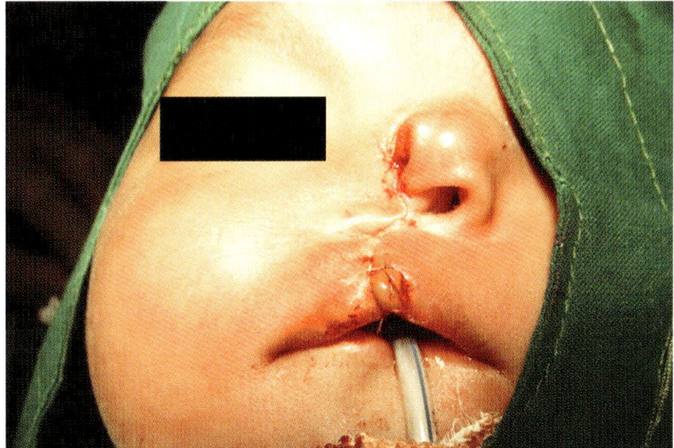

**Fig. 14.5:** Repaired with Millard's rotation and advancement method

## NUMBER 5

There is a vertical soft tissue deficiency between the lateral portion of the lip and the lower eyelid cleft.

## NUMBER 6

There is soft tissue furrow radiates from the oral cammissure towards the lateral two third of the lower eyelid.

## NUMBER 7

There is cleft extending from angle of mouth laterally and superiorly towards the preauricular hairline causing macrostomia. The maxilla is hypoplastic and clefting is through pterygomaxillary junction with hypoplasia of the alveolar process producing a posterior open bite (Figs 14.6 to 14.11).

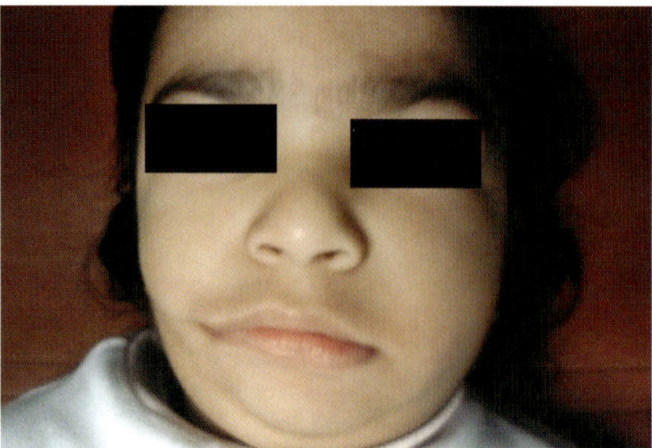

**Fig. 14.6:** Right number 7 cleft: macrostomia

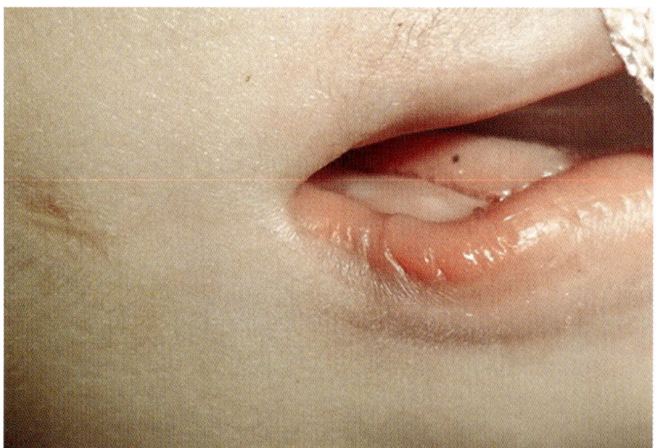

**Fig. 14.7:** Right number 7 cleft macrostomia

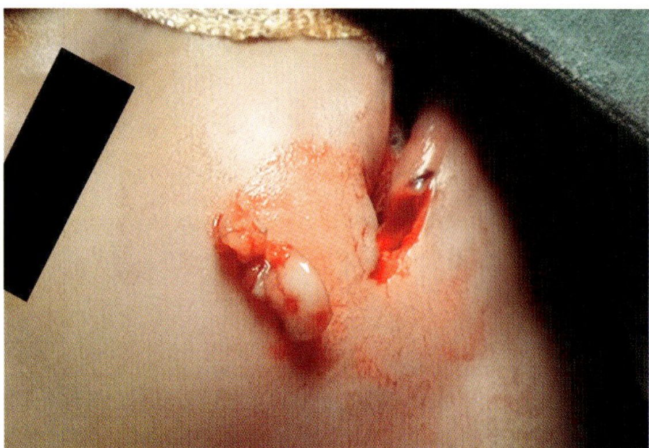

**Fig. 14.8:** Angle of mouth is created at mid-pupillary line extramucosa, and soft tissue is excised

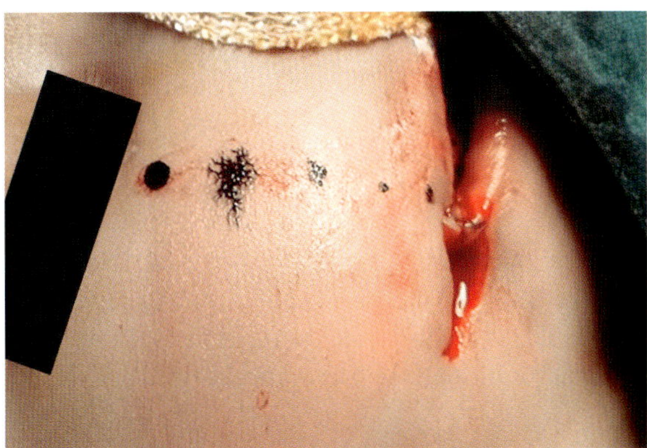

**Fig. 14.9:** Lip mucosa is sutured with 4-0 vicryl

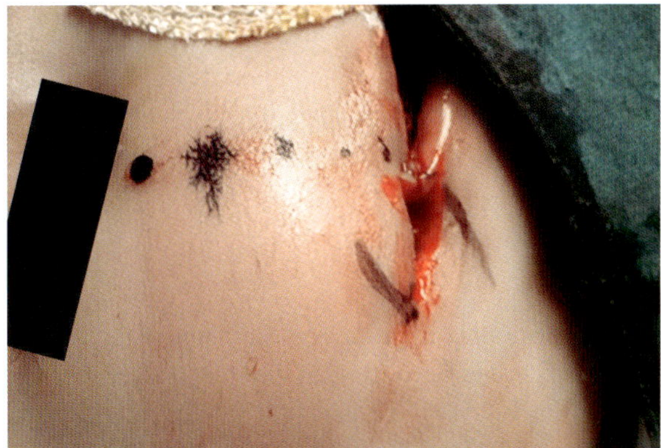

**Fig. 14.10:** Z-plasty is planned for skin closure

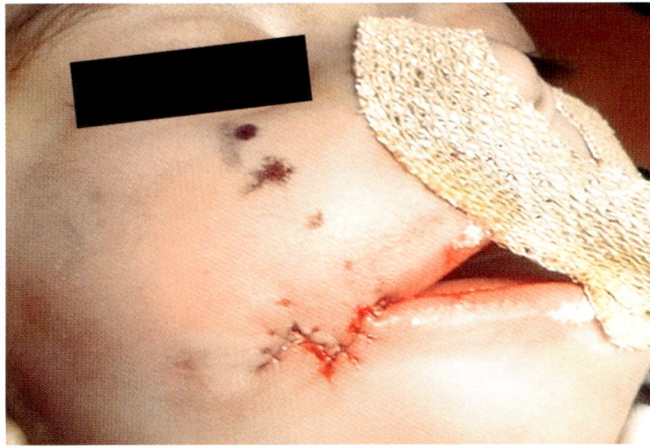

**Fig. 14.11:** Z-plasty completed

## NUMBER 8

There is soft tissue deformities of the mouth, auricle and periorbital tissue. There is bony deficiency of orbit over lateral aspect.

## NUMBER 9

There is superolateral bone deficiency of orbit causing lateral displacement of the globes. Outer canthus and lateral third of upper eyelid are distorted. There is asymmetric hypoplasia of the greater wing of the sphenoid with associated posterior and lateral rotation of the lateral orbital wall.

## NUMBER 10

There is elongation of palpebral fissure with bulb displaced inferiorly and laterally. A broad frontal encephelocele bulges forward.

## NUMBER 11

There is cleft of the medial portion of the upper eyelid and irregularity of the medial portion of upper eyebrow and tongue like projection of the frontal hair line into the forehead.

## NUMBER 12

There is lateral displacement of the inner canthus with irregularity of the medial end of the eyebrow. There is flattening of frontal process of maxilla, laterally bowing of the medial orbital wall causing orbital hypertelorism.

## NUMBER 13

There is cleft extending medial to the undisturbed eyebrow to end in a short paramedian frontal widow's peak.

## NUMBER 14

There is severe orbital hypertelorism with broad flattening of the glabella and lateral displacement of inner canthi.

## REFERENCES


1. Bradley JP, Kawamoto HK. Rare craniofacial clefts. In: Grabb WC, Smith JW, (Eds). Plastic Surgery. Philadelphia: Saunders. 1990;2922-73.
2. Kawamoto Jr HK. The kaleidoscopic world of rare craniofacial clefts: order out of chaos (Tessier classification). Clin Plast Surg. 1976;3:529.
3. Kawamoto Jr HK. Rare craniofacial clefts. In: McCarthy JG, (Ed). Plastic surgery. Philadelphia: Saunders. 1990:2922-73.

4. Tessier P. Anatomical classification of facial, cranio-facial and latero-facial clefts. J Maxillofac Surg. 1976;4:69.
5. Van der Meulen JC, Mazzola R, Vermey-Keirs C, et al. A morphogenetic classification of craniofacial malformation. Plast Reconstr Surg. 1983;71:560.
6. Allam K, Wan DC, Kawamoto HK, et al. The spectrum of medin craniofacial dysplasia. Plast Reconstr Surg. 2011;127:812-21.
7. O' Rahilly R, Mueller F. Interpretation of some median anomalies as illustrated by cyclopia and symmelia. Teratology. 1989;40:409-21.
8. Sperber GH. Craniofacial Development. Hamilton: BC Decker, 2001.

# Index

*Page numbers followed by f refer to figure*